Prai

Leaf crops produce the most nutrition from the least space while requiring the fewest inputs. The trouble is...many valuable leafy vegetables are unknown to gardeners. Nor do we know how to prepare or preserve them. Dave Kennedy's *Eat Your Greens* provides all this information. The book should be on the shelf of every serious gardener.

— Steve Solomon, Author *The Intelligent Gardener* and *Gardening When It Counts*

Kennedy's new book is a practical instructional manual on how to grow and prepare leafy edible plants, many of which are unavailable at grocery stores and farmers markets, overlooked by gardeners and rarely considered in the kitchen. It offers a simple, grassroots solution to help counter the immense public-health burden that has arisen from our high-calorie, nutrient-poor diet. Reading this book could change lives, communities and society for the better.

— Sean Clark, Professor and Farm Director, Berea College

David Kennedy makes a compelling case for home gardens as a vital element of our food system and for expanding our food and garden horizons by growing super-nutritious greens, including some novel leaf crops and traditional crops used in new ways. A great resource for those wishing to increase their food security, *Eat Your Greens* offers detailed information on growing, eating, and preserving greens that both novice and experienced gardeners will welcome.

— Susan Littlefield, Horticultural Editor, National Gardening Association

Low-fat or low-carb? Vegan or paleo? Whole grain or gluten-free? Nutrition has become complicated by competing diets and health claims. The world's biggest food corporations add to this confusion and profit from it at the same time. In *Eat Your Greens*, David Kennedy cuts through the fog and shows us that the journey to optimum health can begin with a single, simple step into the backyard vegetable garden. The message of why and how we can eat more fresh, nutrient-rich greens isn't a marketing ploy designed to bolster some company's bottom line. It's a timeless, universal truth and one that Kennedy tells convincingly.

—Roger Doiron, Founding Director, Kitchen Gardeners International

Eat Your Greens is a refreshingly thoughtful and practical book for the new wave of savvy gardeners interested in exploring the full potential of home gardens. One of the world's experts on leafy green crops opens his garden gate to show us an amazing array of 21 beautiful and some little-known greens that will make you wonder where they've been all your life. In addition to the directive "Eat Your Greens" we can now add "Read *Eat Your Greens*" as excellent advice that will make us healthier and happier.

— Anita Courtney, M.S.,R.D., Chairperson / Tweens Nutrition and Fitness Coalition

Our work is with the poorest of the poor in developing countries and David's training resources have made the greatest impact on what we do but at the same time I have painfully watched the effects of nutritional poverty in the west for years. Everything that I wished could be said to my western friends is in this new book. There is now no excuse to be destined to a life of mediocre health.

It may be hard to believe but a couple of small four by eight foot kitchen gardens, that take minutes a day to maintain can turn the tide of deteriorating old age for so many reasons. Read the book more than once.

— Dale Bolton, Founder and Director of Organics4Orphans.org

Increase the biodiversity of your diet and your garden by expanding the variety of leaves you eat; often from the plants you are already growing for other uses—even cover crops! If you have heard of eating leaves of some plants, but are hesitant to try them because you have also heard they may contain irritants if not properly prepared, let David Kennedy show you the way. Kennedy's expertise and passion for creating a healthy population with the help of leafy greens are evident in this book. In this ever-changing world we need to stay open to the possibilities of all our gardens have to offer. Great book!

— Cindy Conner, Homeplace Earth,
author *Grow a Sustainable Diet* and *Seed Libraries*.

eat *your* greens

eat *your* greens

The Surprising Power
of Home Grown Leaf Crops

DAVID KENNEDY

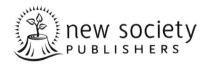

new society
PUBLISHERS

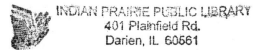

Cover design by Diane McIntosh.
Italian Chicory Basket © iStock (Torquetum)

Printed in Canada. First printing September 2014.

New Society Publishers acknowledges the financial support of the Government of Canada through the Canada Book Fund (CBF) for our publishing activities.

Paperback ISBN: 978-0-86571-751-0   eISBN: 978-1-55092-567-8

Inquiries regarding requests to reprint all or part of *Eat Your Greens* should be addressed to New Society Publishers at the address below.

To order directly from the publishers, please call toll-free (North America) 1-800-567-6772, or order online at www.newsociety.com

Any other inquiries can be directed by mail to:

New Society Publishers
P.O. Box 189, Gabriola Island, BC V0R 1X0, Canada
(250) 247-9737

LIBRARY AND ARCHIVES CANADA CATALOGUING IN PUBLICATION

Kennedy, David, 1947–, author
Eat your greens : the surprising power of homegrown leaf crops / David Kennedy.

Includes bibliographical references and index.
Issued in print and electronic formats.
ISBN 978-0-86571-751-0 (pbk.). — ISBN 978-1-55092-567-8 (ebook)

1. Edible greens. 2. Edible greens — Preservation. 3. Vegetable gardening. 4. Organic gardening. 5. Cooking (Greens). I. Title.

SB339.K45 2014   635'.3   C2014-904442-9
                                         C2014-904443-7

New Society Publishers' mission is to publish books that contribute in fundamental ways to building an ecologically sustainable and just society, and to do so with the least possible impact on the environment, in a manner that models this vision. We are committed to doing this not just through education, but through action. The interior pages of our bound books are printed on Forest Stewardship Council®-registered acid-free paper that is 100% post-consumer recycled (100% old growth forest-free), processed chlorine-free, and printed with vegetable-based, low-VOC inks, with covers produced using FSC®-registered stock. New Society also works to reduce its carbon footprint, and purchases carbon offsets based on an annual audit to ensure a carbon neutral footprint. For further information, or to browse our full list of books and purchase securely, visit our website at: www.newsociety.com

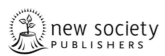

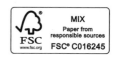

Contents

Part IV: Looking Ahead

Acknowledgments

Special thanks to three people for their help with this book:

to Keith Wilde for the illustrations

to Dan Feather for help with photographs
and other graphical aspects

and to my dear partner Therese Hildebrand,
who worked hard on every part of the book.

Introduction

We have become deeply confused about food. Cooking shows are now more popular than cable news shows—even though we now spend less time actually cooking than ever before. The average supermarket has doubled in size over the past 15 years and now carries over 38,000 items.[1] Americans eat roughly 20 percent of their meals in cars. On average, we eat about 200 pounds more food per year, including 56 pounds more meat, than we did in the 1950s. Two thirds of American adults are overweight, as are nearly one third of the children. Half of the overweight population is clinically obese, despite the $40 billion a year we spend on weight-loss programs and products.

What's going on? Where are we headed? In another 15 years will grocery stores have 70,000 items? Will we eat *half* our meals in cars? Will we eat *even more* meat? Will we all be too fat to move? The simple answer is no. We are beginning to reach saturation points for many of these consumer trends. For example, the sale of bubbly soda, among the worst of all our foods, has gone flat, gradually declining over the past seven years.

The Law of Diminishing Returns will eventually impose itself on our food system. Initially, adding new items to our supermarket shelves provided the excitement of novelty and the benefit of greater choice. However, the relative benefit of adding more items begins to decline at a certain point until there is no further benefit to adding more choices for shoppers. Beyond that point, the chore of making ever-more decisions outweighs the value of increased choice.

One hundred and fifty years after the introduction of the McCormick reaper, the modern food miracle is becoming a drag. The thrill is gone. New food products flood our cultural landscape, but we can only greet them with a fraction of the exuberance we showered on Tang and TV dinners. Despite the frantic efforts of an overheated persuasion industry, there is more genuine enthusiasm for raising chickens in backyards than there is for new fast food menus.

No longer confined to the counterculture, dissatisfaction with our modern food system is creeping into the mainstream. A preference for locally grown food sold through locally owned stores and restaurants is emerging within the key demographic of young, affluent, well-educated consumers. The big supermarket chains had little trouble incorporating the whole grains, organic produce, yogurt, tofu, and granola that were once found only in alternative health food stores and food co-ops. There is nothing about "organic" that makes it inherently out of bounds for global corporations. But the same is not true for "locally grown" and "locally owned." These terms can offer the shopper useful information about not just the product they are buying, but also about the process that produced it.

Throughout North America, farmers markets are flourishing as more consumers yearn to actually meet the farmers who grow their food. Between 1994 and 2012, the number of farmers markets in the US has grown from 1,755 to 7,864. New farmers markets are now opening at a rate of over 700 a year.[2]

Another interesting trend is the growth of Community Supported Agriculture (CSA). CSAs are systems that link (generally, small) farms with consumers who pay an annual subscription fee to receive weekly boxes of produce. The CSA concept was introduced in Japan in 1965 where it was called *teikei*, or roughly "food with the farmer's face." For the CSA farmer, planning and marketing are simplified because the crops are pre-sold. For the consumer, the draw of the CSA is often as much about making a meaningful connection with a local farmer as it is about getting fresh produce. The exact number of CSAs isn't known, but there are hundreds of new ones forming each year.

Despite this impressive growth of both farmers markets and CSAs, only the most determined and resourceful "locavores" can get all their food from within the area surrounding their communities. Only the most optimistic among them believe that high-quality, locally produced food will drive industrially produced food out of their towns. The high hurdle keeping local foods from once again becoming our primary source of nourishment is the stark economic reality that the industrial system produces and distributes an abundance of food cheaply.

An industrialized farmer can now produce roughly 12 times more food in one hour than his counterpart could in 1950. The increase in farmer productivity has given us a reliable supply of cheap food. It has also allowed (or forced) almost all of our population to move away from the farms and pursue other forms of employment.

Critics of the industrial food system and local food advocates rightly point out that some of this huge increase in productivity is an illusion. Some of that increase is actually the result of transferring or "externalizing" production costs in the form of soil erosion or contamination of water supplies with agricultural chemicals. The industrial method of food production has also benefited from government largess, mainly in the forms of crop subsidies, subsidized crop insurance, and tax-supported research at state universities.

Increasingly, North Americans have two antagonistic food systems. The dominant system—controlled by a small handful of corporations—grows food on large monoculture (single crop) farms. It then processes that food in factories, and sells it through chain supermarkets and restaurants. The incipient local food system is trying to offer consumers a smaller amount of higher-quality food produced in a more sustainable and neighborly manner. There is little reason to think that either system will triumph completely and eliminate the other. More likely, people will begin to cobble together a new hybrid food system by combining elements of each.

This book proposes adding a third leg to this hybrid food system, one that addresses some of the limitations of both the corporate and the local systems. That leg is a re-envisioned home vegetable garden movement with a greater focus on leafy vegetables. Too often, the home garden is seen as no more than a weekend hobby in the realm of suburbia or perhaps as a nostalgic throwback to a simpler era. I am convinced that the home kitchen garden and the checkerboard plots of community gardens are poised to become an integral part of this embryonic hybrid food system. Grounded in sound science and economics, the home kitchen garden will be a useful and instructive component of a complex modern food system.

Because home grown vegetables and fruits don't have to be sold, they are free from most of the mind-numbing calculations of cost and price that control what crops get grown and how they are grown for both the largest and smallest of commercial farms. Many of the brightest new farmers see their love of growing food devolve into an obsessive and oppressive effort to earn a living in the small gap between their production costs and the price for which they can sell their food. Despite the real differences in the corporate and local models of the food system, both are ultimately shaped by the unrelenting need to create more space between cost and price. Without these constraints, home kitchen gardens are much more able to integrate beauty, curiosity, relaxation, and other vital human values into the food-growing experience.

Home gardens are on the cusp of explosive growth in productivity. A new wave of savvy gardeners is beginning to explore the full potential of the home garden. Increasingly, they are realizing that by doubling the size of the garden, doubling the depth of the soil, doubling the percentage of organic matter, doubling the length of the growing season, and doubling the nutritional value of a harvest, they can dramatically increase the productivity of their non-mechanized labor. Unlike the productivity leaps of industrial agriculture, these gains can be made while improving nutrition, biodiversity, and local control.

Growing leaf crops in kitchen gardens specifically addresses the inability of industrial agriculture to provide good nutrition, adequate biodiversity, and meaningful local participation. Home grown leaf vegetables are potentially the most nutritious, most bio-diverse, and most local of all foods. This book explains how to realize that potential.

Leaf crops produce more nutrients per square foot of growing space and per day of growing season than any other crop. They also have more nutrients per calorie than any other food, especially the nutrients commonly lacking in our diets. Given that 69 percent of Americans are overweight or obese, this vitally important. There are over 1,000 species of plants with edible leaves. Some part of this largely untapped food resource can thrive in almost any situation.

Table 1 gives you a glimpse of the surprising nutritional power of some of the non-traditional leaf crops described in this book.

This book shows how familiar garden plants such as sweet potato, okra, beans, peas, and pumpkin can be grown to provide nutritious, edible leaves as well the better-known tubers and fruits associated with those plants. This strategy enables us to harvest significant amounts of additional protein and energy from our leaf crops. It also explains how to improve soil by growing edible cover crops.

In this book, you will learn how to grow 21 spectacular leafy crops, how to extend their harvest, and how to preserve them for year-round use. You will learn how to make leaf concentrate—perhaps the most nutritious food on the planet—from your own garden. A selection of original recipes shows you how to incorporate all these beautiful greens into delicious meals.

Table 1. Nutritional Power of Some Non-Traditional Leaf Crops

Fresh Leaf 100 grams (about 3½ ounces)	Vitamin A RAE (Retinol Activity Equivalents)	Iron mg (milligrams)
Lettuce	25	0.4
Cabbage	5	0.5
Chaya Leaves	1167	5.8
Grape Leaves	1376	2.6
Moringa Leaves	378	6.7
Toon Leaves	1550	8.7
Wolfberry Leaves	1407	9.5

Leafy vegetables are great foods, but they are not miracle foods. They won't make us brilliant, or charming, or pain-free. Growing more high-quality greens in home gardens certainly won't resolve all of the many inadequacies of our globalized food system. However, I hope this book convinces you that you personally have some real power to improve our food systems and that growing leaf crops in home gardens is an excellent place to begin.

PART I

Balancing Our Food System

1

Two Out of Three Cheers

❖ ❖ ❖

The Power of the Industrial Food System

Most food in North America is supplied through a global industrialized network. Food produced and distributed through that industrial system is cheaper now than it has ever been in human history. Just 15 minutes, working at the US minimal wage, can earn the money needed to buy enough food to meet a person's daily requirements for calories and protein. Of course, this would not be gourmet dining, and not everyone has a job, even a minimum wage one. There are numerous other problems, including high housing, medical, and transportation costs, as well as the usual spectrum of social, emotional, and educational factors that can keep a person from getting the food they need. However, the high cost of basic foods isn't one of them.

In 2011 Americans spent less than ten percent of their disposable income on food, and nearly half of that was spent eating away from home. Sixty years earlier, food made up nearly a quarter of the entire household budget in the US. This is about the same percentage that Mexicans now spend. In many countries, such as Pakistan and Kenya, half of all income goes to buy food. Despite the increasing productivity of industrial agriculture, the appallingly unequal distribution of the world's resources results in roughly one billion people still falling asleep hungry most nights. Few of them live in North America.

It is not simply a plentiful supply of staple foods that North Americans enjoy. Food remains cheap even as we eat our way up the food chain. As people used to say, we eat "high on the hog." That is, we eat a lot of luxury foods with high nutritional value, especially meat, fish, milk, and eggs. These foods of animal origin require greater resources to produce than plant-based foods and, as a result, they are almost invariably more expensive. Still, North Americans generally have enough income to fully indulge their taste for animal-based foods. In fact, only the half million people living in tiny Luxembourg eat more meat than Americans.

Our food prices may fluctuate a bit from year to year, but even through droughts, freezes, floods, and wars, we have a reliable supply of nutritious food. This dependable source of nourishment affords even average citizens luxuries like pursuing higher education, diverse careers, and the arts. The constant availability and low cost of food is so central to our modern way of life that it is easy to take it for granted.

Food Systems

There are basically four interconnected parts to any food system: production, processing, distribution, and consumption.

Production

The vast bulk of our food begins as wide swaths of single crops growing in neat rows on huge farms. Growing large areas dedicated to a single variety of plant is known as *monoculture* or *monocropping*. In North America, corn and soy are by far the most dominant of our food crops—in both acreage and sales—followed by wheat. Farmers growing these monoculture crops have tried to remain profitable chiefly by increasing yields while decreasing their labor costs.

Crop yields, especially of corn and soy, have climbed steadily over the past 80 years, primarily through the increased use of soluble fertilizers, irrigation, and specially bred seeds. During this same time, herbicides and insecticides were also introduced. By reducing competition from weeds and insects, they allowed much more food to mature and reach the market. The combination of these techniques has led to per acre corn yields six time greater than what they were in 1931. Similar, if not quite as dramatic, improvements were made in the yields of other food crops.

Agricultural labor costs have been minimized by some of the same techniques that increased yields. Using concentrated fertilizers to stimulate growth and replace lost soil nutrients requires far fewer hours of work than maintaining soil fertility with animal manures and cover crops. Spraying herbicides to control weeds takes far less time and sweat than repeatedly hoeing them by hand or even cultivating them with a tractor. The labor required to control weeds has recently been even further reduced by the introduction of seed that has been genetically modified to survive specific herbicides. Nearly 90 percent of all corn and soy in the US is now grown from genetically modified (GM) seed, and most of it has been engineered for herbicide resistance.

During the same time that per acre corn yields jumped six-fold, the average farm size in the US nearly tripled—to 418 acres. Canadian farms grew, too, to an average of 778 acres. With two and a half times as much land to tend, farmers turned to bigger machinery to keep their labor costs low. Taken together, this combination of larger farms, bigger machinery, concentrated fertilizers, herbicides and pesticides, irrigation, and improved seed has made the North American farmer incredibly productive. Today's farmer can produce as much food in four hours as his counterpart in 1950 produced in a 48-hour work week. This amazing 12-fold leap in labor productivity underlies much of our modern food system.

Coinciding with the explosion in corn and soy yields came a transformation in raising livestock. Concentrated or Confined Animal Feeding Operations (CAFOs) began in the 1950s as a new way to raise poultry more profitably. Large numbers of animals were fed in confined areas where their movement was very limited. Adapting the strategy of the assembly line, the CAFOs scaled up, streamlined, and mechanized the process of raising farm animals. This allowed them to speed production, create a more uniform product, and simplify processing and sales—all while sharply reducing labor costs.

The principles of factory livestock farming were soon extended to cattle and swine, and even to raising fish. The US produces roughly the same amount of pork as it did in 1950, but just eight percent as many farms are needed to match that output now that the CAFO model is dominant. Despite some consumer resistance, the bulk of our meat and eggs is now produced with this method. Because the confined animals are not able to forage or graze for any of their food, everything they eat needs to be brought to them. All of the different types of animals are fed concentrated diets comprised mainly of corn and soy. Thus the success of the CAFO model depends upon an enormous and cheap supply of those two field crops.

Processing

The mountains of corn, soy, and wheat and the enormous herds and flocks of cattle, pigs, and poultry that leave the farm are just the raw material for making our food. The food processing industry turns this torrent of raw farm produce into chicken nuggets, milk shakes, school lunches, linguine Alfredo, and virtually every other thing we eat. Even though almost all the food we eat is processed in some way, processed food has a bit of an image problem. Processing is sometimes seen as a set of marketing tricks used to turn wholesome "real" food into irresistible concoctions of starches, sugars, oils, and an unholy slew of chemical additives. And while it is true that a large and profitable segment of the industry does indeed churn out "junk food," food processing provides some important benefits to our society. Industrial food processing makes our foods clean and convenient. Unlike many people in the world, we don't need to carefully sort through a bag of rice or beans to pick out pebbles or moldy seeds. Industrial machinery does that for us. It also removes bones, peels, grinds, juices, filters, sifts, dries, cans, freezes, pre-cooks, weighs, and vacuum-packs our food. All of this leaves us with a very convenient supply of food. Our food is not only the cheapest in human history, it takes the least time and effort to prepare for eating.

As with agriculture, economies of scale and industrial analysis have dramatically lowered the per unit cost of almost all food processing. Specialized machines, such as 100-horsepower extruders can make uniform food products quickly (try to make Cheerios or Pop Tarts at home by hand). Because the specialized processing machinery is very expensive, huge volumes of food must be processed in one place in order to justify the initial investment in equipment.

Distribution

After this mountain of industrial food is grown and processed, it must then be distributed to the hundreds of millions of homes where it will eaten. This is obviously a daunting logistical challenge. The average bite of food eaten in the US has traveled at least 1,300 miles. Generally, the farther food travels, the greater the number of people who have role in getting it to the table. When food is imported from another country (and an increasing percentage of our food *is* imported), the number of customs officials, inspectors, brokers, freight consolidators, and shippers involved is impressive.

There are certainly advantages to getting the food you need from nearby, but what are the benefits of an industrialized global food distribution system? The most obvious is that you can eat things that don't grow where you live. That may include oranges, bananas, chocolate, coffee, salmon, avocados, and a range of other distant delicacies. Secondly, foods that do grow where you live might not be growing when you want to eat them. For many people in the Northern Hemisphere, apples in May, tomatoes in November, and spinach in August are foods that fall into this category.

A third advantage of shipping foods long distances is that they can be grown by the lowest-cost provider. For instance, large, highly mechanized farms in California have climate and soil conditions that are advantageous for growing carrots. A local grower with less-than-ideal soil and weather can't compete on price with big California operations like Bolthouse Farms, which processes six million pounds of carrots a day. The economic advantages are so significant that one third of all the produce grown in the United States comes from California's central valley.[1]

In order to ship food 1,300 miles and still make money, the cost of both the food and the transportation has to be kept very low. Industrial-scale agriculture and food processing produce the low-cost food, and inexpensive fossil fuel keeps transportation costs down. The global food distribution system weaves together ocean cargo routes with automated ports. Free trade agreements that allow multinational companies global access to the lowest-cost food providers are essential to the economics of this system. So is sophisticated technology. From the farm where it was grown or from its port of entry, most food continues its journey in trucks. Customized computer programs match up extensive national highway systems with regional warehouses and link those warehouses to the retail stores.

To the average person, the colossal distribution web that binds them to the industrial food supply is largely invisible. Only when the food arrives on the shelves of our supermarkets or on the table at a local restaurant do we become aware of its existence.

The embrace of information technology is one of the defining characteristics of the industrial food system. Nowhere is this more evident than in food distribution. Bar code readers in the check-out aisle of supermarkets not only tell customers how much to pay, they tell store managers how much of what products have sold that week and what needs to be reordered. Store discount cards increasingly track consumer data, which allows food mar-keters to identify and influence shopping trends. When you hit your favorite pizza place on speed dial and they answer the phone knowing your name, address, and your preference for green olives, that's information technology distributing your food. When the pizza arrives hot at your door in 30 min-utes or less, that is the industrial food system providing you convenience.

Consumption

Ultimately, the most important step in any food's journey takes place when it is eaten. Americans each eat about 2,000 pounds of food a year. So, when someone makes a New Year's resolution to not eat a ton of food this year, it is not hyperbole. We now each eat about 200 pounds more food per year than we ate in 1980, so it's not surprising that the pants feel a bit tight.[2]

How we consume food shapes how the entire food system is organized. For Americans, convenience rules. For example, Americans spend about 30 minutes a day preparing food, compared to an average of 52 minutes for peo-ple in other industrialized nations.[3] The percentage of our food dollar spent on meals away from home nearly doubled from 1970 to 2000, and that trend is continuing.[4] With estimates of nearly one in five meals being eaten in cars, it is not surprising that food companies are designing soup that fits into car cup holders and bacon and egg breakfasts that can be eaten with one hand while driving.

The final—and often ignored—step in food's trek is as *waste*. The indus-trial food system is reasonably good at avoiding waste on the front end. Farmers, slaughterhouses, and processors have found many ways to make economic use of by-products that were previously thrown out. Packing house wastes are often used to feed animals, and the blood and bones re-maining from slaughtering meat animals is turned into fertilizers and food for other animals. Where things get sloppy is on the retail end. Where things get really bad is where the food is meant to be consumed: our homes. Our food waste per person has nearly doubled since 1974. Astonishingly, as much as 40 percent of all food produced in the US is now wasted.[5]

Flaws in the Industrial Food System

Unless you live in the Amazon rain forest or a deserted lighthouse, you have probably heard some of the less-than-glowing reviews of the industrial food system. Some of these criticisms are essentially the flip side of what supporters of the predominate system consider to be strengths. For instance, the tremendous output per man-hour keeps food costs low, but it's also a major cause of unemployment. The reliable consistency and uniformity of industrial fare benefits the consumer, but at the expense of lost flavor and variety.

Ultimately, the most damning judgment against the industrial food system is that it cannot be sustained. Critics state the obvious: complete dependence on non-renewable energy sources is not a recipe for long-term sustainability. Many go on to point out that industrial agriculture is also losing its topsoil far faster than it can be rebuilt. Actually, the average rate of soil erosion on large monoculture farms has declined since the 1970s and appears to have leveled off. While definitely an improvement, the rate of erosion is still about ten times greater than the rate of natural soil formation.[6] This is hardly a strategy for a durable food system.

The lack of biological diversity is another significant problem for industrial agriculture. Most biologists agree that maintaining a large number of unique genetic possibilities is important to the sustainability of ecosystems in general and the food system in particular. The lack of diversity is present both on individual farms, where monocultures are the rule, and throughout the food system as a whole. The aggressive promotion of a few profitable hybrids and genetically modified seed varieties is leading to a widespread and permanent loss of traditional and heirloom varieties of food crops. It is estimated that over 90 percent of the historical genetic diversity of our food crops has been lost since the advent of industrial agriculture; some well-documented studies show that up to 98 percent of vegetable varieties in the US have been permanently lost in the past 100 years.[7,8]

Perhaps the most vexing concerns about the industrial food system relate to the nature of the food itself. The industrial food system generally does a much better job with quantity than with quality. This is especially true with nutrition. Overall, the industrial food system supplies far too much refined carbohydrates, fats, and salt, with far too little fruits, vegetables, and whole grains. This results in diets with too many easily absorbed calories, and with shortfalls of certain protective vitamins, minerals, and antioxidants, as well as fiber. This industrial diet has been blamed for sharp increases in the rates of obesity and diabetes.

A lot of ink and air time has been expended on these issues, but here's a depressing summary:

• 36 percent of American adults are obese. 69 percent are overweight.[9]

- Obesity raises annual medical costs by $2,741 (in 2005 dollars) per person.[10]
- In addition to medical costs, the epidemic of obesity also costs society in the form of more food, more clothes, more fuel, bigger furniture, lost work time and output, and weight control programs.
- The number of people diagnosed with diabetes has risen from 1.5 million in 1958 to 18.8 million in 2010, an increase of epidemic proportions. People with diagnosed diabetes have average medical expenses of about $13,700 per year.[11]
- Mexico has now surpassed the US in per person soda consumption and has become the world's fattest nation. They have passed a tax on soda to try to slow the avalanche of medical costs from obesity and diabetes.

Another (increasingly vocal) criticism of the industrial food system is leveled at the inhumane treatment of cattle, swine, and poultry in crowded feeding operations. A small group of animal rights activists initially called our attention to the way animals are treated in the CAFOs. As graphic images of crowded animals in factory farms reach more eyes, the number of people put off by the factory farms swells. Industrial meat producers have generally responded to this unease not with better living conditions for the animals, which would have significant costs for them, but rather with greater restriction of access to the CAFOs—so people can't take more pictures.

Lastly, there are concerns that the global industrial food system is damaging the social and economic fabric of local communities. Some degree of autonomous control over the food supply is considered by many planners to be essential to the health and resiliency of local communities. The vast economic power of the global food corporations makes it difficult for small communities to have more than a passive consumer-oriented input into how they eat.

What Is the Take-Home (or Take-Out) Message?

We want our pizza delivered fast and hot. We see the industrial food system like a dazzling blind date. We are drawn to its obvious attributes, but the more we learn about it, the more we become aware of its flaws.

Can we have healthier food that is still cheap, appealing, and always available? Can we grow food in a way that is sustainable while holding on to the huge gains in productivity? Well, yes, and no. Some possible improvements are pretty obvious. Reducing the sugar and salt content in processed foods would be easy and relatively painless. More whole grains could be brought to market without changes in farming techniques because refined grains are, of course, made from whole grains.

Highly processed foods with 25 or more ingredients could be simplified. Foods targeted to children could be held to a higher nutritional standard. Shipping foods that are mostly water, such as fruits, vegetables, juices, and milk, long distances doesn't make sense if those foods could be locally produced.

We have arrived at the point where we need to analyze the entire industrial food system, component by component. Then we can fully consider the merits and drawbacks of alternative approaches from an informed and pragmatic viewpoint. Only then we can begin assembling and testing hybrid food systems to find what best meets the often-conflicting needs of people and the planet.

For the first time in human history, overeating is a larger global threat to our health than hunger. As tedious as trying to lose weight may be, most of us would rather wake up with that problem than with the older one of not having enough to eat. It is time to offer up congratulations and a toast to those who have, over centuries of hard work, replaced hunger with plenty. It is likewise time to graduate to the new task of producing that plenty more sustainably, with greater justice, respect, and beauty. In short, with more grace.

This food is the gift of the whole universe—
the earth, the sky, and much hard work.
May we live in a way that is worthy of this food.
May we transform our unskillful states of mind, especially that of greed.
May we eat only foods that nourish us and prevent illness.
May we accept this food for the realization of the way
of understanding and love.

« THICH NHAT HANH »

2

Less of the Same?

❊ ❊ ❊

The Promise of the Local Food System

The Local Food Movement

Widespread and growing disgruntlement with the industrial food system has begun to coalesce into a very loose-limbed movement that is dedicated to creating alternative ways of meeting our need for food. Especially in Europe, the US, Canada, Japan, and Australia, this dissatisfaction with the status quo is being expressed through the emergence of several locally focused food-distribution schemes. Sometimes "local" is defined as foods grown, processed, and eaten within a somewhat arbitrary radius of perhaps 50 or 100 miles. Often, the term "local food" simply describes food distributed directly from the producer to the consumer, rather than through a long-distance supply chain. Two of the most important and fastest growing elements of this local food movement are farmers markets and community supported agriculture (CSA).

Farmers Markets

Farmers markets are retail markets where farmers sell their produce directly to the consumers. This is hardly a new concept, but after a long gradual decline, farmers markets are experiencing an extraordinary renaissance. In 1994 there were 1,775 farmers markets in the US. By 2012 there were over four times that number. Farmers markets in the US typically have between 10 and 100 vendors. Most markets are held outdoors, once or twice a week during the peak harvest season. About 15 percent of the markets in cold weather areas continue to operate through the winter by going indoors.

19

Most farmers markets offer some minimally processed local foods, such as breads, cheeses, and jams, along with the fresh fruits, vegetables, and meats. Some markets also have locally made craft items. It is common to have some restrictions on what can be sold. For example, many markets prohibit reselling food that was bought elsewhere at wholesale, and some require that all items come from within a set distance from the market.

Community Supported Agriculture

Community supported agriculture is a newer idea for marketing farm produce. It began in Japan and Europe in the 1960s as a way of spreading the risk of farming between farmers and consumers. Cities were expanding, and prime agricultural land was being quickly lost to residential developments. Much of the original motivation of the community supported agriculture movement was to protect the farm belt around towns by shielding the farmers from some of the unpredictability of the real estate market. By the 1980s, the concept had taken root in North America, starting in the northeast and the Pacific coast.

The basic idea of the CSA is the formation of a partnership between the farmer and the consumer. Typically, consumers subscribe to buy a share in a farmer's crop, thus assuring their access to fresh produce and sparing the farmer some of the risk and trouble of marketing. In a good year, consumers receive baskets bursting with produce. In years when conditions conspire to damage the crops (perhaps through drought, flooding, or freezing), consumers get baskets that are less bountiful, and so share any loss with the farmer.

Because the subscription payments are usually made before planting begins, the farmer can more accurately estimate how much of each crop to plant. The pre-sale of the crop provides the cash that farmers need for seeds and supplies at the beginning of the growing season. It also allows the farmers to concentrate on growing superior quality food with fewer worries about marketing during their busiest season.

There are dozens of variations on the community supported agriculture strategy. Many CSAs are joining together to offer customers a wider variety of food in their weekly baskets. For instance, a vegetable farm might combine their products with those from a dairy and egg farm, or a grass-fed beef farm. There is no doubt that the CSA phenomenon is spreading rapidly. However, there is no standardized definition of a CSA farm, nor is there a reliable means of counting them. Estimates of the number of CSA farms in the US in 2012 range from about 4,000 to about 6,000.

Core Beliefs

These two marketing schemes, farmers markets and CSAs, share a core set of beliefs that defines the local food movement. These beliefs fall roughly into four overlapping categories that describe the benefits of local food: nutritional, social, economic, and environmental.

Nutritional Benefits: There is nearly unanimous agreement within the local food movement that fresh, minimally processed food is healthier than highly processed food shipped in from afar. This opinion is generally supported by nutritional science. There is also widespread (but not unanimous) support within the local food movement for the idea that organically grown food is more nutritious than its conventionally grown counterpart. Mainstream nutrition science is somewhat less convinced on this point.

Social Benefits: The local food movement holds it as self-evident that face-to-face interaction between producers and consumers of food will strengthen community trust and cohesion. In addition, farmers markets supply opportunities for farmers to talk with other growers about agricultural problems that are specific to that area. Shoppers quickly realize the markets offer social possibilities beyond simply getting fresh food. People come to listen to street music, line up child care, drink coffee, hire workers for odd jobs, leave messages for each other, and casually engage in dozens of other social activities. Advocates for local food are convinced that these informal webs of social interactions help build and maintain civic vitality.

A second social benefit of the local food movement can be found in the rejuvenation of the status of the "farmer" in our society. Compared to conventional farmers (who grow commodities for large-scale supply chains), the local farmer is about 14 years younger, twice as likely to be female, Hispanic, or African American, and twice as likely to have a college degree. Local farmers tend to be especially interested in environmental issues, well-versed in agro-ecology, and are likely to see local farming as a calling rather than as a source of income. Mercifully, the cultural deriding of farmers as naive ill-informed rubes, hayseeds, and hee-hawing bumpkins in overalls seems to have finally run out of steam. After nearly a century of decline, both the social status and the number of farmers is beginning to rise again, buoyed by the growth of smaller, more local farms.

Economic Benefits: The local food movement promotes the concept of resilience over the raw efficiency of scale. The resilient economy has a complex network of many small producers and distributors (who are often the same people) rather than dependency on a few huge food corporations. While the global food system can stabilize supply by drawing from different climate zones, the local system uses a very different model of resilience. As an example, the global system would quickly import apple juice from China to fill a shortage caused by a drought in Pennsylvania. Local food advocates take a longer-term view. They want to make sure that when the rains return, the local apple growers haven't been driven out of business because they can't compete with cheap Chinese apple juice. Their approach prefers trying to resolve local food production problems to managing the volatility of foreign labor markets, international trade agreements, and currency exchange rates. Keeping food supply lines as short as possible with the minimum number of middlemen increases community control over the food it eats.

Advocates often cite the *multiplier effect* as a major benefit of localizing food. The multiplier effect posits that money spent on locally grown food tends to circulate locally, generating jobs and income within the community. In contrast, long-distance shipping of food that could be locally produced depletes the local economy because money goes to distant owners. Few argue the potential of this effect to improve depressed local economies, but most of that potential won't be realized until the local food systems become much larger.

Environmental Benefits: How the local food movement views environmental issues closely parallels the concept of economic resilience. A patchwork of smaller farms growing a wider variety of crops is closer to the ideal of a stable ecosystem than are the 1,000-acre monocrops of corn and soy. Soil on smaller local farms is more often protected through the use of animal manures, cover crops, compost, and crop rotations. These are considered the best practices for building and maintaining soil fertility and structure.

Local farmers are also far more likely to employ best practice Integrated Pest Management (IPM) techniques that are much gentler on the ecology of the area. People shopping for local food expect that the land producing that food is well cared for and that local farm animals are treated humanely. The agro-ecology perspective of local growers combined with high expectations of local consumers creates strong motivation for environmentally sound food production.

Flaws of the Local Food Movement

Critics often suggest that local food can't compete with mainstream industrial foods on price, availability, or variety. They often see local foods as a solution mainly for an elite of relatively wealthy, well-educated people. They don't see how local can be scaled up enough to provide an adequate and affordable source of food for low-income people. The most dismissive critics see the local food movement as a passing fad, soon to join the ranks of disco, urban cowboys, and mood bracelets.

Are Local Foods Too Expensive? The perception that local foods are more expensive than industrial foods is quite widespread and persistent. The reality is not that simple. Several studies have contradicted that idea, claiming that the prices at farmers markets and supermarkets are very similar, especially when organic produce is compared. One study done in California concluded that farmers markets routinely have lower prices than supermarkets for similar produce.[1]

Debate over the price of local foods sometimes hinges on what metrics are used. For example, a well-publicized 2010 study showed the cost of obtaining calories from healthy fruits and vegetables to be significantly higher than getting the same number of calories from less healthy refined grains, sugars, and fats.[2] This applied to both locally grown and industrially grown foods. Healthier foods being more expensive than less healthy foods has become a common explanation for the fact that the diet of most Americans falls far short of government health recommendations.

However, local foods rarely include the low-cost processed foods that are highest in refined carbohydrates and added fats and sugars. These are the cheapest source of calories, but far from the cheapest source of many essential nutrients.[3] Because local foods are weighted heavily toward fresh and minimally processed fruits and vegetables, they are very competitively priced in meeting almost all nutritional needs, except for calories. Given the obesity crisis in North America, the benefit of foods that are cheap sources of calories but lack other nutrients is dubious at best, while the benefit of cheaper fruits and vegetables is very significant.

In theory, reclaiming the fat slice of the food pie that currently goes to an assortment of processing and distribution middlemen should make direct-marketed foods less expensive than food sold through longer supply chains. In practice, economies of scale plus a handful of logistical advantages make it hard for local food to compete with industrial food on price. Industrial producers tend to pay less for agricultural inputs than local growers because they buy in much larger quantities. Where the small-scale local farmer is at the greatest economic disadvantage, however, is not in buying supplies, but in per unit labor costs. Tending a thousand acres in one crop is much cheaper *per acre* or *per pound of produce* than growing several different foods on four acres. Profits from larger monocropped farms justify the cost of specialized labor-saving machinery.

Similar economies of scale exist on the food distribution side. The huge volumes involved in the industrial system have spawned sophisticated computerized logistical frameworks for organizing the sale and transport of food throughout the world. As a result, the cost of marketing is much lower *per carrot* for the commodity farmer selling 2,000 tons of carrots than it is for the local farmer selling 200 pounds.

Are Local Foods Inconvenient? From a consumer perspective, the biggest drawback of local foods may not be higher prices but lower convenience and availability. Modern shoppers have become accustomed to levels of availability and convenience undreamed of 50 years ago. Many supermarkets are now open 24 hours a day nearly every day of the year. At the largest supercenters, shoppers can get their groceries, do their banking, have an appointment with a doctor, and get new tires for their car without leaving the store. In contrast, farmers markets and CSAs are typically open only for a few hours once or twice a week during the harvest season. A small percentage remain open during the winter, but they tend to have a pretty limited selection of food.

It is not just the convenience of the supermarkets that consumers have grown accustomed to. They also have become enamored with the convenience of the foods within those stores. Microwave popcorn, frozen pizza and Kung Pao chicken, instant soup, ready-to-eat macaroni and cheese—these are the foods of a people in a hurry. The average time Americans spend cooking has been dropping for 40 years, even as the average number of meals away from home has been rising. Neither of these trends plays to the strengths of the local food movement. Most of the foods available through farmers markets and CSAs require some degree of preparation greater than setting the microwave timer.

Can the Local Food Movement Support Its Farmers? As a rule, local farmers are not adequately paid for their work or for the risks that they take. In addition to the work and risk involved, local farmers must also provide significant resources in the form of land and equipment. Based on either hourly wage or annual income, local farmers rarely make as much money as most of their customers, and not infrequently they fall below official poverty levels.

Local farmers often have an ideological or emotional investment in the idea of being a good farmer; they see what they do as something between a job and a mission. After a few years of very hard work and very low pay, though, the romance of being a farmer often wears thin. The commitment to take good care of the land and to produce the highest quality food all while keeping prices accessible to their customers puts many local farmers into a form of self-exploitation.

This problem is real for growers selling through farmers markets or through CSAs. The CSA structure eliminates some of the risk and some of the long hours of sitting at a booth trying to sell produce. However, even with CSAs, the financial rewards of local farming rarely put a farmer into the same income bracket as her customers. A 2012 study in Massachusetts concluded, "We find that current share prices of CSA farms do not reflect all of the costs of production, and hence might not be an economically viable approach to sustainable agriculture if CSA farms continue their current pricing strategy."[4]

The study suggested that most customers would accept higher prices and that this might make the model more economically feasible for the farmer. Of course, raising prices would also reinforce the idea that local foods are only for the wealthy and thus would probably shrink the pool of potential future customers. Shrinking the pool of customers is not something the local food movement can afford to do if it is to be a serious player in the way we eat. The most damning critique of the local food movement is that it is just too small to make any difference. Current estimates are that only about one half of one percent of food in the US is directly marketed from farmers to consumers.[5] This means that the movement could bring in 20 times more customers and still only make up 10 percent of the total food market.

Are Local Foods Really Any Better for the Environment? There have been a few critics of the local food movement who have questioned the widely held belief that localizing the food system would benefit the environment.[6] For instance, it has been claimed that lamb flown from New Zealand into England had less negative environmental impact that locally raised lamb. Most of the environmental advantage of the New Zealand lamb derived from the fact that the British lamb was fed grain, whereas in New Zealand the lamb was raised in pasture. This was a reasonable indictment of feeding meat animals grain, but unfortunately ignored the best environmental option—that of local grass-fed lamb. Similar studies have shown that importing tomatoes from warmer climates uses less fuel than growing them in heated greenhouses over the winter. Of course, you could easily argue that fresh tomatoes all winter may be an environmental extravagance regardless of how or where they are grown.

A more interesting criticism claims that local foods may actually consume *more* fuel than industrial-scale food. The local food movement has popularized the concept of counting "food miles" to gauge how environmentally sound a food is. While it seems obvious that getting foods from nearby would require less fuel than getting food from far away, this may not always be the case.[7] Dozens of relatively inefficient pick-up trucks hauling a few hundred pounds of produce 15 miles to a farmers market may actually end up using as much fuel per pound of produce delivered as a much larger truck hauling 40,000 pounds from California.

It is also worth noting that nearly half of the total fuel used in the food system comes from consumers driving to and from markets. In theory, this suggests that driving frequently to small local markets could use more fuel than driving less frequently to supermarkets that carry a wider range of products.

A factor to consider in comparing the overall environmental impact of the two food systems is that the industrial system has spent the past 60 years streamlining to reduce costs, while the local alternative is much newer and still finding ways to minimize its ecological footprint. For the industrial food system, the level of environmental impact is determined largely by the profitability of large-scale mechanized operations. The local food system, on the other hand, has a strong ideological preference for environmentally sound practices. The far greater level of active participation in the local food system is already beginning to generate new responses to these environmental problems. Farmers are experimenting with ride sharing, mobile farmers markets, and biodiesel production for small delivery vehicles.

What's Next for Local Foods?

The local food movement is certainly a long way from being able to supply a significant portion of our national food needs. However, it is relatively new, and it's growing fast. Its supporters are passionate, energetic, and well-educated. Furthermore, the profound failure of the dominant food system to seriously address nutrition and sustainability issues creates openings for the local alternative.

Some supporters have argued that the local food system is a social good that should receive government support to help it grow. Government intervention into market dynamics is always a slithery proposition, but the overused metaphor of leveling the playing field may be more palatable. Providing the local food system with government support similar to what is given to the industrial food system might not exactly level the field, but it could make the climb less steep for local foods.

Some of this is already happening in the form of government-subsidized food-purchasing programs, such as SNAP (Supplemental Nutrition Assistance Program); WIC FMNP (Women, Infants, and Children Farmers' Market Nutrition Program); and the (SFMNP) Senior Farmers' Market Nutrition Program. These programs are rapidly being integrated into farmers markets and even CSAs. The amount of SNAP benefits redeemed at farmers markets increased by 55 percent between 2010 and 2011.[8]

Non-profit organizations, increasingly joined by local governments, are creating programs to support both their local agriculture and the health of their low-income citizens. For example, Chicago's Experimental Station is working with local and state government to implement Illinois' Double Value Coupon Program by including it in the state budget (see experimental station.org). Michigan's Double-up Food Buck and Boston Bounty Bucks in Massachusetts are other examples of non-profits working with government (see doubleupfoodbucks.org and thefoodproject.org/bountybucks).

These programs allow more low-income families to benefit from the more nutritious food available from direct markets and more low-income farmers to benefit from increased sales. This is an area where governments, both federal and local, might realize significant savings from modest investments. The health care costs of diet-related chronic degenerative diseases are staggering. There are always genetic and other factors in the onset of these illnesses but statistically, poor diet plays a very large role. Anything that improves the diet of low-income families would greatly lower government health care expenditures.

The government could also help strengthen the local food movement by providing more funding for agricultural and food technology research that is targeted to smaller operations and to organic growing methods. The spectacular increases in productivity in industrial agriculture are in no small part due to government funding of research at the big land grant universities. Most of this research has been focused on large-scale production, and it has left the local food movement with a research and development disadvantage.

Better use of emergent information technologies could make local foods more competitive. Many modern shoppers prefer the convenience of using credit or debit cards to buy food, and the fact that few farmers markets or CSAs accept cards turns away some potential customers. Experiments with using point-of-sale credit card readers in farmers markets show this would be a very popular addition and would increase sales. There are now several innovative strategies being tried to enable farmers markets to take advantage of consumer preference for credit cards.

The local foods movement is also adopting more sophisticated ways to communicate with potential customers about availability and price. Various permutations of Internet and cell phone apps can provide up-to-the-minute posting of information to farmers market and CSA customers. Before heading to the market, one can now check to see if there is broccoli or if Farmer Joe still has that great deal on peaches. Recipes for unusual items like amaranth greens or Jerusalem artichokes or shallots can be posted to help customers expand their culinary horizons while helping farmers make a decent living.

Another area where the local food movement is trying to leverage computer savvy into sales is with online food delivery services. Retail behemoths Amazon and Walmart are already staking claims to this rapidly growing segment of the $450 billion US grocery business, and many others are joining the fray. However, the convenience of ordering food online is being taken in a different direction by enterprises such as Freshpicks. This Chicago area company supplies its customers with locally grown organic fruits and vegetables, free range chickens and eggs, and grass-fed beef and lamb. The Freshpicks website (www.freshpicks.com) even provides information on which farm grew each item in the delivery basket. This model, which is being adopted by several smaller companies and larger CSAs, offers the customer convenient top-quality food while supporting local farmers.

At this point, local food is far more important as a cultural phenomenon than as an economic reality. Still, whether the focus is on culture or economy, the local food movement is a very dynamic entity. Linear economics tell most of the story of industrial foods, but it is fascination with idea of integrating deeper cultural values into our economy that powers the local food movement. Because it is growing and changing so fast, the best analysis is necessarily only a snapshot of the movement at a given time.

The local food movement won't drive the industrial food corporation out of business anytime soon. Neither will it disappear in our culture's rearview mirror like VHS cassettes or fins on cars. We have industrial food because it is cheap and convenient and available, and we want that. Local foods are a growing part of our life because we want them. That wanting is deep enough for us to overlook some glitches and uneven development. Bumping into friends while leisurely strolling through the farmers market and chatting with the folks that just picked the nutritious vegetables you are buying is simply too compelling a vision for a harried and alienated culture.

We have neglected the truth that a good farmer is a craftsman
of the highest order, a kind of artist.

« Wendell Berry »

3

Away from the Market

✻ ✻ ✻

Raising Food, Not Money

If you view the struggle between the local food movement and multinational food conglomerates as a David-and-Goliath story, where would the humble home kitchen garden fit in? It would hardly be a footnote to the story about transformations in the food system. The average farm in the US is about 30,000 times larger than the average kitchen garden. How are kitchen gardens *not* trivial to changing the food system? In many ways, kitchen gardeners are the flip side of the industrialized food system. From this position, they may shine a light on that system and suggest some necessary changes.

Who Gardens?

Home gardeners are an incredibly diverse bunch of people. For example, in the US, a nation with over 312 million people, 43 million households grow a food garden.[1] That is a large group of people engaged in small-scale agriculture. In contrast, there are one million farmers in the US. While the acreage and tonnage of food involved in home food gardening is minuscule compared to commercial farming, the combined experience, creativity, and diversity of this human resource is vast. While only 14 percent of farmers are female, more than half of all kitchen gardeners are women. African Americans and Latinos are also far better represented among gardeners than within the ranks of commercial farmers.

While farming is almost necessarily a rural activity, gardening happens not only in rural areas but also in suburbs, small towns, and even in poor neighborhoods of densely populated cities. Innovative organizations such as Grown in Detroit, a cooperative of 37 of the city's market gardens; Growing

Power in Milwaukee and Chicago; Jones Valley Urban Farm in Birmingham; and BUGS in Baltimore are revitalizing the idea of the urban Victory Garden. Some of the inner city food gardening programs emerged as a response to the recognition of "food deserts." The Quesada Gardens Initiative in San Francisco offer the local youth an alternative to drug and gang culture. Some try to address both the cost of food and common health concerns. For instance, Projecto Jardin is a community garden in East Los Angeles that combines growing nutritious food with growing herbal medicines.

The demographics of kitchen gardeners also favor upwardly mobile trendsetters; scientists, artists, engineers, professors, designers, architects, and entertainers. Cities with large universities, high-tech jobs, and a tolerant, culturally diverse population tend to have vigorous community garden programs—with waiting lists of enthusiastic gardeners. Even the White House has a kitchen garden; and Michelle Obama's enthusiasm has helped get dozens of urban and school garden projects started.

The new wave of kitchen gardeners is increasingly connected through the Internet; there, growers can select from thousands of plant varieties and dozens of seed catalogs from all over the world. Gardeners can now quickly find online help identifying the insects that are eating their crops and how to stop them. Video clips showing gardeners how to make raised beds, build cold frames, or transplant seedlings can greatly accelerate their progress from novice to expert.

Why Do They Garden?

What kitchen gardens bring to the food system extends beyond the diversity and connectivity of its gardeners. In addition, the motivation behind home gardening is fundamentally different than that of farming. Farmers are almost invariably motivated by earning money. They may have other considerations, but they grow things to sell. To earn more money, farmers can either grow more, sell what they grow for a higher price, or reduce the cost of growing it. They rarely have enough clout in the market to affect price, so they try to grow more food and reduce the per unit cost of growing it. Both of these efforts have resulted in larger and larger farms.

Home gardeners, on the other hand, are rarely trying to earn money selling the food they grow. They have other motivations. The National Gardening Association's large study *The Impact of Gardening in America* (2009)[2] lists the top 11 reasons given for growing a home food garden (gardeners could choose more than one reason).

- To grow better tasting food (58%)
- To save money on food bills (54%)
- To grow better quality food (51%)
- To grow food I know is safe (48%)
- To feel more productive (40%)
- To spend more time outdoors (35%)
- To get back to basics (25%)
- To have food to share with others (23%)
- To live more locally (22%)
- To have a family activity (21%)
- To teach my kids about gardening (30%)

Note that three of the top four reasons given for kitchen gardening are to grow food that tastes better, has better quality, and is safer. The implication of this, sometimes explicitly stated, is that many people think that commercially available vegetables are lacking in flavor, nutrition, and safety.

Generally speaking, flavor and nutrition both benefit from freshness, and garden produce is the freshest available. Levels of volatile nutrients such as vitamin C, folate, and other B vitamins begin declining immediately after harvest. While commercial produce typically takes a week or more to get from the farm to the table, garden produce is often harvested immediately before being prepared and eaten.

The particular variety of a given fruit or vegetable can also have a dramatic effect on its flavor and nutritional value. Commercial varieties of fruits and vegetables are chosen mainly for their profitability. This often comes down to high yield, attractive appearance, easy harvesting, good shipping qualities, and long shelf life. Unfortunately, none of these attributes correlate very strongly with good flavor or high nutritional value.

Not intending to sell their produce gives home gardeners the luxury of being able to choose among dozens of varieties that are exceptionally tasty or especially rich in certain vitamins and minerals. Not only can home gardeners choose varieties of common vegetables that are more flavorful and nutritious, they can also grow unusual plant species that are not usually available in supermarkets.

One might assume that food sold commercially would be safer than food grown in home gardens because of the various health inspections and permits required. This is not always the case. Food grown in the home garden is usually handled only by one or two family members—people who have a strong personal stake in the safety of that food. It is still possible to get food-borne infections from dirty hands, contaminated compost ingredients, or animal feces, but those infections are usually very localized and self-limiting.

The same is not true of the commercial food system. A 2012 outbreak of listeria (*Listeria monocytogenes*) food poisoning was traced to a single contaminated batch of fresh spinach. The spinach was recalled from stores in 15 states. Such outbreaks are actually relatively common by-products of a highly centralized food system. In addition to listeria, the past few years have seen widespread outbreaks of food poisoning caused by salmonella, *E. coli*, and hepatitis A on mass-distributed lettuce, spinach, peppers, cantaloupes, tomatoes, and green onions. And these are among the very fruits and vegetables we are advised to eat more of for better health! But a contaminated bunch of spinach coming out of a kitchen garden can't sicken people living thousands of miles away.

Food poisoning is not the only safety concern that home gardeners have with commercial produce. An increasing percentage of gardeners choose to grow their crops with organic methods in order to avoid eating food with pesticide residues. Despite reassurances that the small amount of residue on conventionally grown produce is not a health risk, much of the public remains wary. Conclusive testing of agrochemicals is difficult and expensive. Unintended long-term negative consequences are always a possibility. Many gardeners and conscientious consumers simply reason that, while the small amount of pesticide residue on their food may not be a serious health threat, they would rather not eat any pesticide at all.

Another concern for some gardeners and potential gardeners is the issue of genetically engineered food.

Until recently, genetically modified crops were mainly used to produce animal feeds and cotton. However, a concerted drive is under way to extend this biotechnology to vegetable seed, and very likely, genetically modified vegetables will soon be showing up in supermarkets and restaurants. The European Union and over two dozen countries require genetically modified foods to be labeled as such, though the US and Canada still do not. Gardeners are able to control what they grow and how they grow it, and many appreciate the ability to exclude pesticides and GMOs.

The Economics of Home Gardening

The National Gardening Association study estimated that, on average, food gardeners spent $70 each year on their vegetable gardens and grew roughly $600 worth of vegetables. (They calculated an average yield of half a pound of vegetables per square foot of garden and an average retail price of $2 per pound.) This may sound like a high figure, but the gardener's vegetables are worth more than the farmer's because they replace vegetables bought at the higher retail price, whereas the farmer sells his vegetables at a wholesale price, which is often less than one third of the retail price.

Getting $530 worth of free food is a good deal. That represents about ten percent of the average family's total yearly food bill. Of course, the vegetables don't just pop up out of the garden. On average, gardeners spent five hours a week working in their gardens. Assuming the garden is in operation for 20 weeks each year, the gardener spends 100 hours, earning $530 worth of vegetables, or $5.30 an hour. This is not a terrific pay scale. In fact, it falls below the US legal minimum wage.

This will not necessarily continue to be the situation. There are several reasons to think that food gardening may be poised to make a leap in productivity, echoing the jump that commercial farmers have made in the past 60 years. By extending the growing season, planting seeds more densely in better-quality soil, using trellises to incorporate more vertical space, and choosing the most nutritious crops, the cost-to-benefit ratio can shift significantly in favor of gardeners. Top gardeners are already getting vegetable yields three times (or more) higher than what average gardeners harvest. In the near future, those kinds of yields may become commonplace.

As a job, home gardening may not pay well, but it is an easy commute to the backyard; there is no clock to punch, and every day is "casual Friday" or "Hawaiian shirt Wednesday." It provides good exercise without the drive to the gym. Gardens are flexible enough to make good use of informal seasonal paid labor (retirees, teenagers on school vacations, etc.). Unlike most low-paid jobs in the food industry, gardening is usually a satisfying endeavor. A television interview with innovative Tennessee gardener, Adam Turtle, offers some insight. Adam was asked, "How much time do you spend in your garden?" Without a pause, he replied: "As much as I possibly can." This is probably not the way most workers in the food industry feel about their work.

Home Gardens and Health

The industrialized food system is spectacularly efficient at supplying calories in attractive and convenient forms, but it does a much poorer job making fruits and vegetables available to everyone at affordable prices. This is exactly where kitchen gardens can shine.

Most government health agencies and independent nutritionists worldwide recommend eating five or more servings of fruits and vegetables every day for optimal health. MyPlate, the new US government nutrition logo, graphically informs us of the relative importance of vegetables in the diet. The risk of heart disease, stroke, high blood pressure, obesity, diabetes, several types of cancer, and preventable blindness are all significantly reduced by a diet rich in vegetables.

Simply put, people who grow gardens eat far more vegetables and people who eat more vegetables have fewer serious health problems, and treating serious health problems is far more expensive than buying vegetables. Several studies have shown that participating in gardening increases vegetable consumption. A study done in Flint, Michigan, by researchers from Michigan State University concluded that, "adults with a household member who participated in a community garden consumed fruits and vegetables 1.4 more times per day than those who did not participate, and they were 3.5 times more likely to consume fruits and vegetables at least 5 times daily."[3] Of greater long-term economic importance is the impact of gardening on the diet of children. One in five American children is now obese. Clearly they are not getting enough help developing healthy eating habits.

There is an emerging consensus that children who experience gardening also eat more vegetables. The early development of healthy eating patterns in children is a critical factor

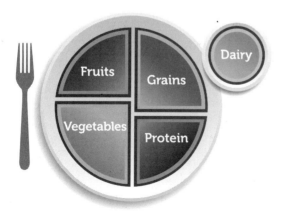

in the effort to reduce future health care costs. In analyzing the results of 20 studies of school gardening and nutrition education programs, researchers from Oregon State University concluded "one striking and robust result emerged: gardening increased vegetable consumption in children, whereas the impacts of nutrition education programs were marginal or non-significant."[4]

Home Gardens and the Health of the Planet

The production, distribution, and preparation of food have more impact on our natural environments than any other human activities. Finding ways to get food without making a mess of the natural world is a pressing need. Home gardens can help.

Kitchen gardens bring two important environmental advantages to a food system. The first is reduced transportation. Hauling fresh produce across continents in refrigerated trucks uses a lot of fossil fuel and contaminates a lot of air with exhaust fumes. A short walk to the kitchen garden is obviously lighter on environment.

The second environmental benefit that gardens bring is biodiversity. Stable natural environments organize themselves as ecosystems with many species interacting in both competitive and cooperative ways. The larger the number of species of different organisms living in an ecosystem, the more likely that it is healthy and stable. Compared to commercial farms, kitchen gardens are havens of biodiversity. Almost all food produced commercially is grown in large monocultures. Monocultures are by definition not biologically diverse environments, and the recent dominance of herbicide-resistant crops has greatly exacerbated the loss of biodiversity from farmlands.

Organic farms are typically smaller and more diverse than conventional farms. Kitchen gardens are smaller still and even more diverse. Most gardeners are growing primarily for home use rather than sales. Because people don't want to eat just one type of vegetable, they grow a much wider variety of crops than farms. These polycultures do a much better job than monocultures at providing key ecological services such as cleaning and recycling air and water, reducing drought and flooding, and providing habitat for songbirds as well as providing a wider range of useful foods and fibers. Homes that have a range of plant life including ornamental plants, lawns, and shade trees sharing space with vegetable gardens are especially diverse.

Also, kitchen gardeners are an important force for maintaining the diversity of agricultural crops. Because commercial agriculture is growing only a small handful of profitable crop varieties, the need to conserve rare and heirloom varieties has become more critical. Seed banks or botanical gardens play an important role in this effort, but often can't provide the complex real-life conditions that allow strong plants to develop. Gardeners can help maintain these heirlooms by growing them in a wide variety of climates and soils. Greater interest in seed saving and increasing awareness of plant genetics among many home gardeners is helping to create and maintain localized vegetable crop varieties.

In a time of smart phones, high-speed Internet and hundreds of channels of television, the pull of the garden is as strong as ever. Kitchen gardens are small, but far from trivial. They are a gift to our children and a tool they will need to create a food system that is healthy, fair, and durable.

Every child should have mud pies, grasshoppers, water-bugs, tadpoles, frogs, mud-turtles, elderberries, wild strawberries, acorns, chestnuts, trees to climb, brooks to wade in, water-lilies, woodchucks, bats, bees, butterflies, various animals to pet, hayfields, pine-cones, rocks to roll, sand, snakes, huckleberries and hornets; and any child who is deprived of these has been deprived of the very best part of his education.

« LUTHER BURBANK »

4

Scaling the Food Mountain

❖ ❖ ❖

Matching the Parts of the Food System to What They Do Best

The first chapters of this book describe three different scales of magnitude within our food system: the global industrial scale, the local commercial scale, and the home garden scale. Developing a durable food system that meets the needs of all the people without damaging future prospects is not simply a matter of choosing the best of these scales. Rather the question is how do we nest these scales within each other so they are all able to perform the functions to which they are best suited.

Ecology Begins at Home

While agriculture was busy mastering techniques to control natural environments in order to pump out prodigious volumes of food, the biological sciences were probing deeper into the nature of those environments. With great patience and ever more sensitive observational tools, biologists have been studying the lifestyles of some of the millions of species of living organisms that share the planet with us. What they are finding is astounding and humbling.

Some examples: Dung beetles use the Milky Way for celestial navigation. Flowers send electrical signals to inform bees of waiting pollen. Plants shape soil chemistry by selectively feeding bacteria and fungi with enticing chemical compounds released from their root hairs. Fungi thrive inside the tomb of the Chernobyl nuclear reactor by using gamma radiation as a food source. So, while growing 200 bushels of corn on an acre of land is certainly an impressive survival skill, other species have learned a few survival skills of their own over the past few billion years.

How the estimated eight million species of living organisms interact with each other and with their environments is the realm of ecology. Applied ecology is a tool that uses ecological principles to make real-life management decisions. It will be an essential tool for producing the food we need without destroying the basis for future food production. As we become better at applying ecological principles to growing food, the simplistic manipulations now basic to industrial agriculture may appear in the rearview mirror as blunt instruments.

Breeding for the highest yields, force feeding soluble fertilizers, and poisoning any plants or animals competing for our crops has been a successful strategy for producing abundant cheap food with little labor. It is unlikely that we can persist in this strategy for much longer, much less expand upon it, to feed additional billions of people. If we are to continue feeding so many humans, we may need a form of agriculture that gives greater consideration to the welfare of non-human species, an agriculture formed around a less anthropocentric world view.

Both inspiration and practical guidance for agro-ecology can come from looking at how mature ecosystems operate. A mature, or climax, ecosystem is a community of plants and animals that has reached a relatively *steady state* and that can run indefinitely on the sunlight that falls on it. Two of the most essential traits of a mature ecosystem are efficiency and diversity. Any effort to incorporate these two attributes into our food system will likely pay significant dividends.

Efficiency

Efficiency describes the amount of useful output compared to the total input in any system. Natural ecosystems tend to make very efficient use of resources. That is, they produce a lot of living tissue relative to the energy, water, and nutrients available as inputs. The only energy source accessible to natural systems is sunlight, but they have had a very long time, sometimes billions of years, to develop and test myriad techniques for optimizing that energy. In many natural systems, for example, fluids are moved using logarithmically or progressively growing spirals, because they are the most efficient configuration. Spiders can spin their webs at ambient temperatures, whereas man has to generate very high temperatures to produce Kevlar, the substance nearest in tensile strength to a web.

In contrast to natural ecosystems, industrial food production supplements available sunlight with massive inputs of energy from petroleum, coal, and natural gas. The profligate use of this supplemental energy has engendered a level of sloppiness that would doom any natural ecosystem. It will also eventually doom any man-made system. Because these fossil energy sources are not renewable (at least not within a realistic time frame for us to use them), a system dependent on them can't be maintained indefinitely. Building a durable food system demands that we dramatically improve the basic efficiency of producing our food, so that the system more closely resembles natural sunlight-driven systems.

The logical first step to improving efficiency is to eliminate the obvious waste and energy leaks in our current system. Reducing waste requires focusing first on reducing our *demand* for food rather than on our current strategy of increasing the *supply*. Sober economists are projecting that demand for food will increase by 70–100 percent over the next 40 years and that food production must increase accordingly. On the other hand, it is also estimated that we now waste 40 percent of all food that is produced.[1] If we were to double food production without reducing the percentage that is wasted, we would then be wasting a quantity of food equivalent to 80 percent of what we are currently producing.

The more rational course is to strip demand down to a minimum and then consider the different possible ways of meeting that demand. This rationale applies to energy policy in general—it makes sense to switch to more efficient light bulbs and vehicles before building new electric plants and offshore oil rigs.

There are many simple ideas for reducing food waste. These include not demanding cosmetically perfect produce in our supermarkets and eating leftovers before they spoil. Composting food scraps and recycling those nutrients back to food-growing land rather than sending them to landfills is another obvious example. But the most fundamental waste in the food system is overeating.

The average American consumes over 500 calories a day more than we did in 1970.[2] The extra calories make us fat and sick and waste over half a pound of food per person per day. Much of this overeating is induced by taunting ads and oversize portions and food with prices too low to pay for its sustainable production.

The most wasteful facet of overeating is the excess consumption of animal products. Meat, eggs, and dairy products require far more resources per calorie delivered than do plant-based products like grains, beans, and potatoes. The most promising way to reduce demand for food is by consuming less meat and other animal products. Estimates of food demand all assume higher levels of meat consumption as incomes rise globally. While grazing animals can make efficient use of sparse and tough grass, most meat is now produced by feeding confined animals grains and soybeans. These grains and beans are far more efficient as foods when they are eaten directly by humans, rather than being first fed to animals and only then converted to food.

There may be some health benefits to eating a small amount of animal-based foods, but the planet cannot support billions of large carnivores. A diet that is 90 percent plant based can more than adequately provide all the nutrients we need, and a completely vegetarian diet is sufficient if some care is taken in choosing foods. Currently, North Americans, Australians, and Europeans consume about 1,000 calories per day of animal-based foods. Moving toward a more plant-based diet would simultaneously reduce the negative environmental impact of the modern diet and improve our health dramatically.

A diet that is 90 percent plant based and 10% animal based would enable a more sustainable and more humane integration of animal rearing into our agriculture. Pastured poultry, along with grass-fed beef and lamb, requires far less energy and water and generates far fewer greenhouse gases and other pollutants than do factory-farmed animals. These more environmentally friendly methods would become more feasible options if our meat consumption dropped by two thirds.

Diversity

Diversity, or variety, at every point throughout the food system helps create resistance to sudden shocks or collapse. The ability of a system to adapt creatively to inevitable change depends on having a large population of possible solutions. This diversity includes the range of organic life in the soil, the number of species and varieties of plants and animals raised, the number and range of sizes of farms and gardens, as well as the number of food processors, distributors, and food vendors.

Redundant suppliers of critical services hedges our bets. Being able to derive essential nutrients from multiple foods is one of the human omnivore's chief survival advantages. Whenever key nutrients come from just a single source, however wonderful, cheap, or delicious it may be, vulnerability arises. When there is a single buyer for farm produce, farmers suffer.

There may possibly be some short-term advantage to having a few huge corporations gain monopolistic control of a sector of the food industry, but in the long run, having more players allows for both more competition and more cooperation, and reduces the abuse of power. Economies of scale in the food system greatly increased productivity, allowing for specialized equipment, uniform processes, and high output. Economies of scope encourage more democratic participation in the food system, allowing for greater variety of products and services, better protection of local environments, and better integration with local culture.

We are all engaged in some part of recreating our food system, whether as a consumer, a farmer, a cook, or a gardener. After we have plugged some of the more obvious leaks in our food system by recycling food wastes and reducing over-consumption, especially of animal-based foods, how can we arrange a food system with enough efficiency and diversity to run smoothly for 1,000 years or more?

An efficient food system would form as a set of nested scales much as natural ecosystems exist in nested scales radiating outward from microclimates to watersheds and continents. Each scale is autonomous and self-regulating but also interdependent with the other, larger ecosystems. In terms of our food system, these scales of production would radiate outward from home gardens, through local small farms, to distant larger farms, and eventually to global suppliers. The home scale offers the greatest level of control with the least transportation needs. Local farms usually have more space available but work within the same climate as the home scale. Larger, more distant farms can take advantage of different climates and economies of scale, such as the use of larger machinery. Global suppliers have very different climates and can provide small volumes of high-value foods, such as coffee, spices, and cacao.

Foods in North America travel an average of over 1,300 miles from the farm to the plate. Most of these food miles are unnecessary and wasteful. As pointed out earlier, the rationale for shipping high-water-content foods like lettuce across the continent is very weak. Fruits and vegetables are typically 85–95 percent water. Grains, legumes, nuts and seeds are usually 5–11 percent water. Obviously, it makes sense to try to grow fruits and vegetables as near to where they will be eaten as possible, whereas it might be reasonable to ship dry rice, lentils, and almonds from areas where they can be more economically grown.

The overall efficiency of the food system would benefit from growing all of our food as close as possible to where it will be eaten. This is eminently feasible with almost all vegetables and many fruits. Upgraded home gardens have the potential to become the primary source for most vegetables, berries, apples, and pears. In addition, they could become significant suppliers of higher-calorie crops like potatoes and sweet potatoes, as well as eggs. Out-of-season crops, especially greens, can often be grown in unheated hoop houses, cold frames, or pit greenhouses with less environmental impact than shipping them cross country.

Beyond the scale of the home kitchen garden or community garden plot, the local commercial farm sector is ready and capable of increasing production. Small, local commercial farmers are an important force for containing urban sprawl and protecting the land surrounding our towns. They are often best suited for producing meat, milk, and eggs in a humane and environmentally sound manner. Decreasing our consumption of animal products and then getting most of what we do eat from local farms would have significant nutritional, environmental, and economic benefits. Local farms can also be the source of fresh fruits and vegetables that are difficult to grow in kitchen gardens.

Moving still further outward from home and local food production, one encounters the industrial scale of agriculture. This scale is perfectly positioned to grow a wider spectrum of staple crops that store and ship well. These big monoculture farms now grow predominately corn, soy, and wheat. Without completely changing their focus from high yields with minimal labor, these farms could fairly easily diversify their plantings to include many other low-moisture field crops.

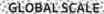

GLOBAL SCALE

**High value foods that cannot be
produced more locally**

Coffee, tea, cacao, spices, smaller amount
of bananas, and other tropical fruits

INDUSTRIAL SCALE

**Large farms, food manufacturing,
chain supermarkets**

Grains, pseudo-grains, legumes, and oilseeds
(wheat, corn, rice, barley, oats, millet, quinoa,
amaranth, buckwheat, soybeans, pinto beans,
chick peas, lentils, sunflowers, Canola, safflower,
etc. Animal feeds and hay for local farms.

Higher nutritional quality processed foods

LOCAL COMMERCIAL SCALE

Small farms, CSAs, farmers markets

Pastured poultry and eggs, grass-fed beef and
lamb, small scale dairy. Most of remaining fruit
and vegetable needs.

Breads, cheese, jams, sauces, etc.

HOME SCALE

**Kitchen gardens, community
garden plots**

Most of our vegetable needs,
much of our fruit, some eggs, etc.

Home canning, freezing, drying,
and fermenting

Barley, oats, rye, triticale, millet, sorghum, and teff are other grains that could be grown on these farms with minimal changes to the specialized equipment. In addition to soybeans, the big industrial farms could also grow a range of high-protein legume seeds, including chick peas, lentils, pinto beans, lima beans, black-eyed peas, and a dozen others. Nutritious pseudo-grains such as amaranth, quinoa, and buckwheat (which are eaten like grains) could also be grown on these farms. Plantings of oil seed crops could also be diversified to include more sunflowers, safflowers, sesame, hemp, and pumpkin seed.

These farms could also support and be supported by the local farms through the sales of supplemental feed and hay for local farm animals. Diversifying their crops and localizing their markets could provide economic benefits to these farmers and ecological benefits to the farmland.

For the sake of efficiency, global foods should be largely limited to small amounts of low-moisture, high-value specialty foods, such as coffee, chocolate, tea, and spices. Shipping large quantities of basic foods around the world because they can be produced a bit cheaper elsewhere is an idea left over from the innocent days before any global warming or environmental awareness.

Most people interact with the food system primarily as consumers. We can certainly become better informed and more discerning consumers, and that is an important piece of building a better food system. We can all make more efforts to get our foods from their most appropriate scale of production. However, only the home garden scale offers opportunities for millions of regular folks to step right into the food system as full participants. Kitchen gardeners can take food through all its stages from seed to table to compost and back again to the table, turning their backyards into healthy food micro-systems.

PART II

Getting Started

5

Leafing Home

✿ ✿ ✿

The Potential of Home Grown Greens

The first section of this book considered some of the strengths and weaknesses of three scales of production within the food system: the dominant industrial scale, the rapidly growing local food movement, and small but widespread kitchen garden scale. It then looked at how these different scales of production and distribution could be nested together to make major improvements in the efficiency and long-term health of our food system.

This section presents the case for growing leaf vegetables in home gardens as a specific way to address several things that the industrial food system and the local small-scale commercial food systems are poorly equipped to do. Leaf vegetables are plant leaves (sometimes including the stems and shoots) that are eaten as food. They are also called *greens*, *potherbs*, *leafy greens*, or *salad greens*. A leafy vegetable patch growing in a backyard garden may strike you as an unlikely place to begin rebuilding a food system. In fact, the green leaf crop is a humble hero patiently waiting for its potential to be unleashed. It is an elemental and underutilized agricultural tool that adapts well to a vast range of circumstance, starting with the home garden.

Why Eat Leafy Vegetables?

Leafy vegetables are good for your health. They are low in calories and full of vitamins, minerals, and antioxidants. The extreme diversity of leafy vegetables presents an interesting variety of flavors, colors, and textures on the plate.

Simply put, leafy vegetables are the antidote to corn syrup in our food system.

In a way, high-fructose corn syrup (HFCS) is the logical conclusion and the ultimate failure of the industrial food system. It begins with the quintessential commodity: government-subsidized genetically modified corn. The corn is shipped to one of 26 corn processing plants in the US, and the starch is stripped from the kernels. This is followed by three stages of enzymatic conversion, then, by various steps involving filtration, ion-exchange, evaporation and blending, resulting in a perfectly uniform product. Just five companies produce 92 percent of this sweetener.

Corn syrup is extremely handy in manufacturing processed foods. It is cheap, colorless, flavorless, and extends the shelf life of many of the diverse products in which it is an ingredient. Because of these attributes, corn syrup is in a lot of products—from soda and pizza to health bars and yogurt. It provides sweetness and calories but none of the protein, vitamins, minerals, fiber, or antioxidants essential to good health. Because it provides energy but nothing else, corn syrup is often described as "empty calories."

The average American eats about a pound a week of high-fructose corn syrup, adding roughly 1,000 of the emptiest of calories to his or her diet. From 1985 to 2010, the price of soft drinks sweetened with HFCS dropped 24 percent, while the price of fresh fruits and vegetables rose 39%. American children took in an extra 130 calories a day from these drinks, while fresh fruit and vegetable consumption remained far below recommended levels.[1] The enormous increase in corn syrup consumption over the past 40 years has coincided with an enormous increase in both obesity and diabetes. It is certainly not the only cause of these two closely linked American epidemics, but neither is the connection mere chance.

A recent study compared the prevalence of diabetes in countries with heavy use of high-fructose corn syrup with that of countries where it is little used, such as Sweden. Even after accounting for being overweight and for total sugar and calorie intake, the rate of diabetes was about 20 percent higher in countries where HFCS was readily available than in countries where it was more difficult to come by.[2]

In contrast to corn syrup, leafy vegetables have deep colors and full, complex flavors. They are rich in a wide variety of nutrients, beneficial antioxidants, and fiber. No other foods can match leafy vegetables for supplying so much nutrition with so few calories. This is ideal for a society where over two thirds of the adults and one third of the children are overweight or obese.

A 2010 study reported in the *British Medical Journal* found that an increase of 1.15 servings of leafy vegetables a day was associated with a 14 percent decrease in the incidence of Type 2 diabetes. No other fruits or vegetables could be linked to a similar decrease in diabetes.[3] The carbohydrates in leaf vegetables are metabolized slowly, so they don't create spikes in blood sugar like refined carbohydrates do. All leaf vegetables have very low glycemic index numbers, and foods with low glycemic index numbers don't contribute to rapid changes in blood sugar levels associated with diabetes and pre-diabetes.

While corn syrup is central to the food processing industry, green leafy vegetables are among the least processed of all foods. Often eaten raw in salads, the only processing necessary for most leafy vegetables is breaking open cell walls to liberate the nutrients within the cell. This can be accomplished with thorough chewing or by blending the leaves at high speed—as is done to make green smoothies. Briefly heating greens also softens and bursts the cell walls because the water inside them turns to steam.

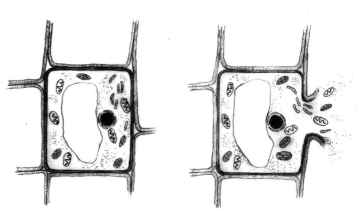

Cell wall ruptured; nutrients released.

Why Grow Your Own Leafy Vegetables?

Of all the categories of food, none is as well suited for growing in home gardens as greens. Because they have a very short shelf life, leaf vegetables are best eaten as soon as possible after harvest. Also, they vary wildly in size, shape, color, texture, and flavor. Not only are different types of leafy vegetables different from each other, they also vary depending on how old the plant is, how warm the weather is, how much rain the leaf crop received, and the fertility of the soil.

The food industry finds the great variability and perishability of leafy vegetables to be problematic. The manufacture of processed foods is predicated on uniform ingredients with long shelf life. Because leaf vegetables are not a predictable commodity, like corn or sugar, they have been largely excluded from industrially processed food. This is part of the reason that Americans eat only about half of a pound of greens a week, despite the unanimous endorsement of nutritional science.

For nutritional and culinary reasons, it is a sound idea to enlarge the role of leaf vegetables in your diet. You can get greens at supermarkets, through farmers markets, or at CSAs. Or you can grow your own. Doing so gives you the best access to the best quality of the widest variety of greens.

Greens are a natural ally of any grower working with limited space. Because they produce more food in less space than any other crop, even a tiny patch of ground dedicated to leaf vegetables can contribute to your diet. For this reason, they have become a favorite in community gardens as well as in backyard gardens. Also, most of the popular leaf vegetables—such as spinach, lettuce, kale, collards, parsley, cilantro, Swiss chard, mustard, and turnip greens—can be easily grown in any container that will hold at least 8 inches of soil. Not everyone is in a position to grow leaf vegetables, but a surprisingly high percentage of people are.

Greens produce more food in less time than any other crop. Some leaf crops, such as amaranth greens, can go from seed to harvest in just 30 days. This means they can be grown in chunks of time far too short for corn or tomatoes or pumpkins. This allows people in places like Calgary or northern New Hampshire, who work with very short growing seasons, to grow some of their own food. For folks feeling hemmed in by cold weather and who are often shut out of gardening, this can be a therapeutic undertaking.

The capacity to produce a large amount of nutritious food quickly in a very small area makes greens the ideal urban crop. For over 60 years, people have been leaving farms and becoming more mobile and urban. Despite the numerous benefits of this migration, many people sense a loss as their schedules become more complicated and unrelated to natural cycles. For these people, the draw of "getting my hands in the dirt" can be strong. Interest in growing food in urban situations continues to rise, and greens are often the easiest and most rewarding foods that can be grown in town. Renters can supplement their diet with the freshest food possible from a few buckets or trays growing leafy vegetables. Greens are even well adapted for growing on urban rooftops, where both weight and space are limiting factors. When the semester ends or the lease expires or the new job in another town comes through, the vegetable garden can be taken along.

It is true that, unless you are pretty hard pressed financially, buying greens is easier than growing them. A few types of leafy vegetables are available at most supermarkets, but no other category of food is as poorly managed by the industrial food system. Most fresh greens are 85–95 percent water, which makes them very perishable. The moment they are cut from the plant, leaves begin wilting, losing both eye appeal and nutritional value. Over 90 percent of leaf vegetables sold in the US are grown in California and Arizona. In order to be shipped, most greens need to be cooled with ice in the field and packed in refrigerated trucks with no delays.

Even this special treatment doesn't give leafy vegetables much shelf life compared to canned beans or flour or cheese doodles or even oranges. For grocers, greens are a lot of trouble. If they don't sell quickly, they look like limp green rags. Profits for food retailers are based on keeping labor costs low, and fresh greens take more labor than simply opening cartons and setting the produce on a shelf. Highly profitable and increasingly ubiquitous convenience stores take this food marketing strategy to the extreme. They have little use and little space for leafy vegetables. If they carry any greens at all, it is only the most popular ones, and many people are fooled into thinking these are their only choices.

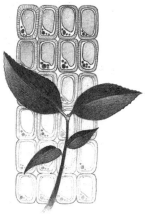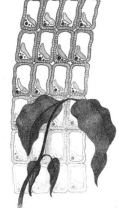

Freshly harvested leaves, wilted leaves.

Though we are repeatedly encouraged to eat more leafy vegetables, industrially grown leafy vegetables aren't always especially good for you. It can be discouraging when you are trying to try to clean up your diet and then you read that leafy green vegetables are responsible for more food-borne illnesses than any other foods. Over ten million Americans become sick each year from eating contaminated leafy vegetables. This represents 22 percent of all the cases of food poisoning in the US.[4] Canadian studies show a very similar pattern; leaf vegetables are also the top vector for food-borne illness there.[5]

Leafy vegetables grown industrially often carry pesticide residues. Lettuce and spinach are both listed in the Environmental Working Group's 2012 "dirty dozen" list of foods with the highest levels of pesticide residues. They also singled out kale for commonly having residues of organophosphate insecticides that have a toxic effect on our nervous systems.[6] It is bizarre that different samples of kale greens, one of icons of healthy eating, showed residues of up to 55 different pesticides according to USDA Pesticide Data Program and the Pesticide Action Network (pesticideinfo.org).

Could these pesticide residues cause health problems? The Environmental Protection Agency tells us they are still safe at these levels. However, it is extremely difficult to test the long-term impact of these chemicals in our systems and to test them in combinations with other common things in our environment, such as fabric softeners, deodorants, caffeine, or antidepressants. Are they safe enough? Who knows? Who wants to find out using their family as test subjects?

Lettuce makes up over 70 percent of all leafy vegetables sold in the US, and most of that is iceberg lettuce. If you were to stay up all night trying to think up the worst food distribution plan possible, you would have trouble coming up with something as illogical as the iceberg or head lettuce industry. While greens as a food category are extremely nutritious, head lettuce is a notable exception. A comparison with kale is instructive. Kale is well known, easily grown, and nutritious (though there are still many greens with greater nutritional value). An equal weight of kale has triple the protein, four times the iron, seven times the calcium, 30 times the vitamin A, and over 40 times the vitamin C supplied by head lettuce.

Growing five billion pounds of a nutritionally crippled food that is 96 percent water in southwestern deserts with subsidized irrigation water is the start of a very bad plan. Then, wrapping each lettuce head in plastic and shipping it thousands of miles in a refrigerated truck doesn't ring of genius either. Days later, the lettuce arrives at supermarkets in areas where local farmers who could be growing far better greens are struggling to stay in business. It sounds like a spoof on modern agriculture, but this is how we eat.

Because it grows close to the soil and is eaten raw, lettuce is one of the most frequent sources of food poisoning. Because it is so mild flavored and tender, it is attractive to many insects and so it must be protected with insecticides. Enough of the pesticides remain on lettuce to make it one of the ten worst foods for pesticide residues. Despite its many nutritional and agricultural limitations, iceberg lettuce is our most important vegetable in terms of sales. You could almost describe it as the corn syrup of leafy greens.

In midst of this somewhat stagnant state of affairs, there is a whiff of change in the air. We appear to finally be getting bored with head lettuce.

The share of sales going to leaf-type lettuce is increasing at the expense of iceberg-head types. We are also gradually becoming more adventuresome, adding a bit of other greens, such as arugula, Asian cabbages, and endives to salads. It should also be noted that leaf vegetables grown with organic methods, whether certified or not, have essentially no pesticide residues. This is true for organically grown greens from industrial farms, local farms, or backyard gardens.

If You Can Afford Organic Greens, Why Grow Your Own?

Buying organic leafy vegetables (along with apples, celery, peaches, strawberries, bell peppers, and grapes) is clearly justified in order to avoid pesticide residues. However, just being labeled "organic" doesn't guarantee that the greens are any fresher, more nutritious, or free from the pathogens that may cause food poisoning. Buying from a farmers market or CSA usually means fresher greens that have been grown in better soil and handled with greater care, but they are probably only available once or twice a week. Buying from either a supermarket or a local food market, your choices of leafy vegetables will be limited by what is most profitable to the retailers or the big farmers.

Growing your own changes all the rules. As you progressively master the craft of gardening, you can gain a level of control over the food you eat and access possibilities well beyond the offerings in the commercial sales outlets. Nowhere are those possibilities greater than with leaf vegetables. There are over 1,000 species of plants that have edible leaves. They offer a dazzling array of shapes, colors, and flavors currently unavailable to consumers.

Leaf crops can be annual herbs, perennial shrubs, or even trees. Some are vigorous twining climbers that can quickly turn a chain link fence into a wall of edible greenery. Barley and Austrian winter peas make mild-flavored greens, and they are hardy enough to last after frost has killed the tomatoes. Cowpeas and fenugreek can be grown for edible leaves and for enriching the soil with nitrogen. They can be planted in between rows of heavy nitrogen feeders, like corn.

Tropical leaf crops can be raised that shrug off the hottest days of summer—when lettuce and spinach turn bitter and go to seed. Summer in much of the world's temperate zones has long stretches of tropical weather. That is all it takes to grow great crops of tropical greens like molokhaya, soko, and vine spinach. When it does turn cold, you can still harvest Siberian kale at temperatures down to 0°F (−17°C). If your soil is too salty for a garden, you can still grow orach, a very salt-tolerant leaf crop in the Atriplex family.

The following chapters will give you the practical information you need to take leafy vegetables to the next level. I hope you can forget all about pale, bland, plastic-wrapped leafy vegetables and have fun taking a plunge into the chlorophylled world of edible foliage.

6

Earthly Paradise

❊ ❊ ❊

Creating Healthy Food Gardens

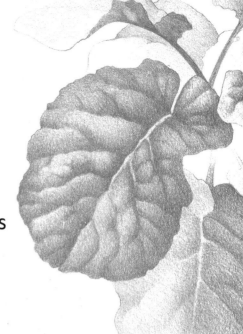

So How Do We Start?

There is plenty of information on how to grow vegetables available to anyone with access to a library or the Internet. Someone new to the field might be taken aback by the sheer number of different ways to garden, many of them pronouncing themselves to be the best. I haven't found the effortless, lazy man's garden that weeds didn't also find. I am unconvinced that there is any can't-fail, foolproof method. Fools are just too persistent to be continually outwitted. Besides, where is the sport in a system that can't fail? How long would we be entertained by a baseball player who hit a home run every time at bat? In my experience, there is no perfect way to grow vegetables, but there are a lot of pretty good ways. And pretty good is a lot easier to live up to.

How do you decide what kind of a garden to plant? Start with where you are and what sort of person you are. A gardener in Seattle or Vancouver needs to have good drainage for all that rain, while a gardener in New Mexico needs to think more about irrigation. What works well in hot, sandy Florida is not the same as what works well in cold, rocky New Hampshire. This seemingly obvious reality is ignored by the authors of many otherwise excellent books on vegetable gardening. It is difficult to speak outside of one's personal experience, and most garden experts have done most of their gardening in just one geographical area.

The same is true with personality. A scientifically oriented person will have trouble with mystical garden philosophies, such as planting by moon cycles. A tidy person may love a square-foot garden for its pragmatic symmetry of neatly aligned rectangular beds. The messy, poetic, or artistic among us might feel restricted or bored by the same garden.

Some of the gardening systems out there are quite rigidly defined, but remember that it is *your* garden. Gardening has been around for so long that most of the currently popular systems are basically just adaptations and modifications of earlier approaches. Freely experimenting with mixing and matching pieces from different schools of gardening can lead to some interesting and useful hybrids. With gardening, enthusiasm often trumps following instructions.

Brokering a peace between the city and the wilderness, gardens offer a miniature template of how we might just be able to get along with the world. The complex interface that gardens create between a person and a place allows for the emergence, albeit on a tiny scale, of uniquely customized terrains. One of the best things about gardens and about gardeners is that no two are alike.

Nothing here is intended to serve as a complete primer on vegetable gardening. There are already many books and websites that serve that purpose well (some of my favorites are listed in the Appendix). In this book, I offer my perspective on some basic elements of kitchen gardening and some practical ideas that have worked for me. By way of disclosure, I am a somewhat chaotic but enthusiastic kitchen gardener who has gardened for over 40 years, mainly in the central Appalachian region of the US. My focus has been largely on edible leaf crops and gardening to improve nutrition.

Elements of kitchen gardening that most gardeners will encounter:

- Site Selection
- Layout
- Soil Improvement
- Starting Plants
- Water
- Weeds
- Pests

Site Selection

Location, Location...: The first step to creating a great garden is choosing a spot. While the home garden is a remarkably adaptable natural canvas for your masterpiece, good garden sites usually share several attributes. Look for a spot that has good access to sunlight, is relatively level, and is as near to your home as possible.

Sunny: Sunlight is indispensable to gardening. In fact, you could think of gardening as a process of using plants to collect solar energy in ways that are useful to you. You can improve poor soil but a shady spot will never make a good vegetable garden. Many plant species have adapted to survive on the thin filtered light of the forest floor. Some of these make good houseplants because the steady temperature and low light intensity inside a house simulates the conditions of the forest understory. These plants survive in the shade, but tend to grow very slowly. Slow growth is not a desirable trait in a vegetable crop.

Try to project your mind through all of the seasons when choosing a spot for your garden. A parcel of land may appear bright and sunny in the early spring when we start thinking about gardens, but it might look a lot shadier after the leaves come out on the nearby trees. Remember also that trees *grow*. It is frustrating when opportunistic trees in your neighbors' yards send roots to feed on the fertility of your garden soil and—even worse—this bonus fertility enables them to send out new leafy branches to harvest the sunlight you had expected to power your garden.

There are a few exceptions to the rule of full sunlight. Access to sunlight becomes more of an issue the farther from the equator your garden is located. The bright overhead sun in the tropics sometimes supplies more light than plants can use, so there, some shade can be beneficial for many vegetable crops. Some crops can thrive in the diffuse sunlight of slightly overcast conditions. In mid-summer, the harvest period of cool-weather leaf crops, such as lettuce, spinach, and kale, can be somewhat extended by providing them partial shade. In most of the temperate zone[1] however, six hours of direct sunlight a day is considered the minimum for good vegetable production, and eight hours or more is preferred. For most leaf crops, heavy shade from buildings or trees will result in lower yields from weakened, spindly plants and more disease problems. Ultimately, it is sunshine that drives plant growth, and shade blocks sunshine.

Level: Land that is level—or nearly level—holds onto water and nutrients better than sloping land. This may help explain why valley people have historically been wealthier than hill people. If the ground has a significant slope, much of the effort you expend improving your garden's soil will wash downhill in a rainstorm. Land with more than a seven percent slope is generally considered unsuitable for vegetable crops. It is certainly possible to build terraces to partially offset this problem. Terraces are level banks for planting with some sort of retaining walls to keep the banks from sliding down the hill. Building and maintaining terraces is very labor intensive compared to gardening on level ground.

Land that is below grade or sunken tends to hold water *too* well. When soil can't drain, it becomes waterlogged, and vegetable roots cannot get enough oxygen for good production. Sunken or enclosed areas with stagnant airflow are more prone to viral and fungal plant diseases. Low spots that are always wet also favor the growth of anaerobic bacteria that generate a unpleasant rotting smell.

Nearby: Choose a spot for your garden as close to your home as possible. You will tend to a garden that you walk through several times a day better than a more distant one. This is the origin of the fortune cookie favorite, "The footsteps of the gardener are the best fertilizer." If you can actually see the deer or groundhog eating your vegetables while you are having breakfast, you are more likely to come up with a strategy to exclude them. You are more likely to stumble out in your pajamas to cover seedlings when frost threatens if the distance to stumble is a short one.

One caution in siting your garden as close to home as possible: be aware of possible soil contamination. Some older houses may have had lead paint and window putty scraped off them which landed in the nearby soil, so it is prudent to site your garden several feet away from older houses.

Community Gardens

People living in rented spaces sometimes assume they won't be able to grow any vegetables. This is often not the case. There are roughly 20,000 community gardens operating in the US, most of which lease garden plots for a small annual fee. The size of community garden plots varies a great deal, with an average of about 300 square feet. Although that's about half the size of the average home garden, it's still more than enough space to grow plenty of intensive crops like greens. Some of the more organized community gardens have classes to help beginners get started. The momentum for creating community gardens is growing as urbanites express their enthusiasm for growing vegetables. In the US, a good resource for learning more (including help with finding a garden near you) is the American Community Gardening Association.

Micro-Paradise: Container Gardens

There are some people who would like to grow a bit of their food but have no space for a garden and for whom a community garden plot is not a good option. Theirs is the realm of container gardening. On the smallest scale of operation, vegetables can be grown in containers. These can be almost anything that will hold eight inches of soil and can be placed in the sunlight for most of the day.

Buckets, old washtubs, beer coolers, kiddie pools, and dozens of other free or cheap objects can be used to grow small greens such as spinach, parsley, cilantro, beet greens, and kale. A hole is a terminal flaw for a water bucket, but that same hole is vital drainage when the vessel is re-purposed as a container garden. Barrels and half-barrels can support larger leaf plants such as chaya or roselle. Some crops, including vine spinach and sweet potatoes, can produce an attractive cascade of edible foliage from hanging containers. These can be used to provide partial shade for windows that would otherwise allow too much summer solar energy into your house.

Water is a finicky concern for crops growing in containers. Because they can't wick water in from surrounding soil, container gardens need watering more often than in-ground gardens. There are several so-called self-watering planters on the market, and I've seen plans for making your own on the Internet. They don't really water themselves, but they do allow for less frequent watering. The Internet has excellent resources on container gardening, though a bit of skepticism is helpful in evaluating them.

Many greens are well suited to container growing because they are relatively small plants with shallow roots. These plants are highly adaptable, fast growing, and produce more food in a given space than most other crops. Even when you have plenty of space, containers can be helpful for keeping sprawling plants like mints or wolfberry from expanding their territory at the expense of your other crops. Gardening in containers can also be a boon to older folks or people with physical limitations because the containers raise the level of the plants and reduce the amount of bending required.

Nano-Paradise: Garden in a Jar

However small it may be, gardeners will find a nearby place to garden. Growing parsley on a window sill or alfalfa sprouts in a jar is still gardening. The principle task is still for the gardener to create conditions in which other useful life forms can flourish. Even if it's raising a crop of yeast to make bread or wine, or a herd of 40 billion lactobacilli to turn milk into yogurt, the urge to grow some of what we eat remains strong, and the gardener will create a place to garden.

Suburban Upraising

Of course, how close to your home you can grow food and how big your garden can be depends on where you live. Historically, towns and cities have been most often located on level coastal and river valley land. Good agricultural land. At the end of World War II, we began turning much of the prime agricultural land surrounding our cities into vast stretches of residential suburban subdivisions. It may not have been the greatest long-term plan, but it happened, and it won't be easily undone.

Besides the conversion of prime agricultural land to housing, there are a few other glaring economic and ecological problems with the suburban model. Houses are too big and too expensive, and too much of the money spent to buy them goes to banks. Since World War II, the size of the North American house has gradually swollen to almost 2,500 square feet, while the size of the household family it has sheltered has steadily shrunk to 2.7 people, providing each of us with more than twice as much dwelling space as what our grandparents comfortably lived in.

The average sales price of new single family home sold in the US in 2012 was $292,200. Almost invariably, new homes are bought with borrowed money. With a typical 30-year mortgage, the actual cost of the house will more than double, with interest payments to the bank making up more than half the total. The banks or lending institutions structure home loans so that most of the early payments go to interest, not principal. Typically, ten years into a 30-year mortgage, the home "owner" has paid off not one third of the loan, but less than one fifth.

Americans move too frequently to fully reap the benefits of land ownership. Economic freedom is a core value, and it has made us a very mobile people. The average person in the US will change his or her place of residence more than 11 times over a lifetime. Most home buyers will re-sell their home long before the mortgage is paid off. This works out nicely for the banks, but is hard on the stability of communities, and it doesn't lend itself to a residential horticulture of stable and productive kitchen gardens. Building really top-quality garden soil generally requires something like 20 years.

Are we ready to give up our suburban way of life? No. But a New Urban movement has been vigorously promoting the infilling of cities and towns to increase residential density for the past 20 or so years. They claim the cultural, economic, and environmental advantages of renovating cities and towns will make us forget all about the suburban dream or what Henry Miller called the "Air-Conditioned Nightmare." Despite some of the fairly compelling environmental and financial benefits of multi-family dwellings, over two thirds of North Americans live in detached single family homes. Most people would still rather live in a place all their own, and this isn't changing. In fact, a recent poll shows that roughly 80 percent of the US population, across most major income, gender, and ethnicity groupings, strongly prefer a detached single family house as their residence.[2]

It is difficult to argue for urban sprawl as a long-term social strategy, but there may be a largely unrealized potential for local foods in the detached single family home plan. Though houses are getting bigger, the average lot size is still about 15,000 square feet (roughly one third of an acre), and this is 12,000 square feet larger than the average house size. This allows plenty of room for a productive kitchen garden. The current average home vegetable garden takes up 600 square feet, or just four percent of the average lot. Should we decide to get serious about local food, we could potentially double the size of our kitchen gardens and still leave nine-tenths of our housing lots for other activities. This is a lot of food production potential tucked away in our residential neighborhoods.

This potential is already beginning to percolate as a modest movement is underfoot to convert at least some part of the ubiquitous American lawn into food gardens. One of the surest ways to judge the traction a movement is gaining is to look at the resistance that it draws. At this point, there is considerable local code enforcement resistance, especially to putting vegetable gardens in the front yard where they are on display and could possibly affect property resale values. Of course, should the new kitchen gardens prove to be popular and functional assets within residential neighborhoods, this could quickly change. The mortgage institutions that actually own the bulk of American homes would likely embrace the newly valuable gardens into building code, not unlike closets in master bedrooms.

There are some shifts in the residential landscape that may foster far greater enthusiasm for kitchen gardens. Beyond an intangible desire to be more connected to the natural world and skepticism about the quality of industrial food, suburbanites are facing some economic realities. High levels of unemployment, job insecurity, and declining real estate values are taking their toll. Over ten million American homes are considered to be financially "underwater," in that they are now worth less than the amount still owed on the mortgage.

The situation has generated a number of grand schemes to save the homeowners. Here's my kitchen garden mortgage rescue plan: Hire young people to convert over-sized houses to duplexes. Having two households share the house and lot would cut mortgages roughly in half. Put in big kitchen gardens to reduce food bills and improve nutrition and health. This might also generate some surplus vegetables and fruit for sharing, trading, or selling through informal local markets.

We are not likely to give up our migratory ways any time soon, but we could take steps to develop a residential horticulture that worked despite our mobility. If kitchen gardens were accorded greater value as long-term investments, it is more likely that they would be passed on like other valuable assets to new people moving into neighborhoods, rather than having garages or tool sheds built on them.

The Internet affords us the ability to keep track of kitchen gardens. Open-source software could be easily applied so that gardeners in town would post and update information about their gardens. Location, soil test results, and crop history of vegetable gardens could be posted online. The data could be correlated with historical rainfall and temperature patterns. Incidence of blights and infestation of pests could be noted. Relatively simple databases could be maintained by county agriculture agents, schools, or garden clubs that would greatly benefit local gardeners. Then people looking to buy a home could see where there are communities of gardeners and which properties have gardens that have been improved over time. This would give the garden an identity independent of the mobile gardeners who worked in it for a while.

Maybe I should run for office.

Locating your garden in a nearby, sunny, and level spot is almost universal garden advice, and it will allow you to bypass many garden headaches. How you lay out your garden and how you prepare the soil are subject to a wider range of opinion and agri-philosophies.

Layout

There is general agreement that you should design your vegetable garden in a way that maximizes planting space and minimizes the need to step on the soil that your vegetables grow in. A system of permanent raised planting beds roughly four feet wide and as long as is convenient has become popular among serious gardeners. The ideal width is determined by the distance the gardener can comfortably reach to work from either side of the bed. Gardeners often opt for four-foot-wide by 25-foot-long beds because they are 100 square feet, which makes calculating seed, irrigation, yield, and so forth, easier.

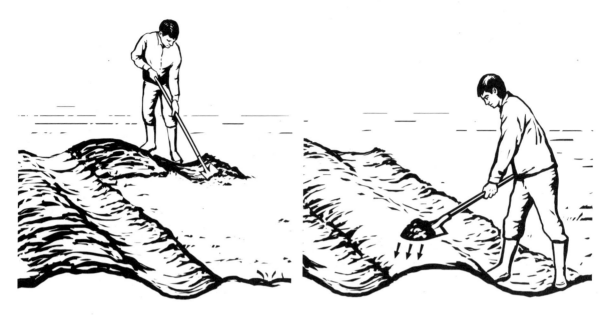

Dig dirt from pathway.   Put it in growing bed.

There are several ways to make raised beds. Most of them involve these two steps:

- Loosening, but not removing, the soil where the beds will be to a depth of about 18–24 inches.
- Removing the top eight inches of soil from what will become the pathways and adding that soil to the bed. This lowers the pathway and raises the bed.

Generally pathways are kept between 18 and 24 inches wide. This width allows gardeners to move freely but doesn't take away growing space from the beds unnecessarily. The soil in the growing bed is improved as described in the following paragraphs and then never walked on again.

The are many advantages of this system over the traditional practice of simply planting vegetables in rows on level ground:

- The ratio of actual growing space to path is much more favorable, resulting in higher yields.
- The soil is deeper, allowing better root penetration.
- The soil in raised beds warms up earlier in the spring, allowing earlier planting of some crops.

- Water and soil amendments can be focused on just the beds and not wasted on walkways.
- The soil in the beds is never walked on; this greatly reduces compaction and allows better soil structure to develop.

The proverbial footsteps of the gardener are only the best fertilizer when they don't compact the soil around the plant roots. Compacted soil allows plant roots less access to the air, water, and nutrients essential to growth.

Traditional row gardens have wide pathways separating long, single rows of vegetables. The rows of vegetables are not normally raised above the level of the pathways. This is a system that was inherited from farming where land was plentiful and labor was scarce. The paths were periodically cleared of weeds by tractors, animal-drawn plows, or rototillers. It is an antiquated form of gardening. Even if you have plenty of space and machinery, no one recommends repeated tillage to control weeds anymore because the damage to the soil structure outweighs the labor benefit.

With home kitchen gardens, space is usually at a premium, and high crop yields are often more important than any savings in labor. These are conditions where the advantage of planting in beds rather than rows is especially desirable. Reliable yield data for vegetable gardens is hard to find because there are a large number of variables and few gardeners are carefully measuring their yields. With that in mind, consider that the University of Colorado Master Gardener Program estimates that beds have an average of five times greater yields than rows and that for smaller vegetable crops, such as radishes, carrots, and greens, the yields from beds may be as much as 15 times greater.[3]

Another obvious and significant advantage of raised beds is that the depth of the topsoil is increased. The effective depth of garden soil is from the surface to that layer of soil that prevents further root growth. Deeper soils can supply more nutrients and water to vegetable crops than can shallow soils. Depth of soil often determines the maximum yield from a crop—especially crops grown without irrigation. While many crops will appear to grow well in relatively shallow soil, they will generally be more disease resistant, more vigorous, and more productive in deeper soil.

Some gardeners put sides up to hold the soil in their raised beds, and some allow the beds to slope gently into the paths. There are a lot of variations on both approaches. The sides tend to make for tidier-looking beds and prevent improved soil from sliding down into the paths. Depending on how sturdy the sides of the raised bed are, they can serve several purposes. Wooden sides are sometime used to secure hoops that can support clear polyethylene sheeting or shade cloth and turn the bed into a miniature greenhouse or shade house. They can also support trellises for climbing plants and keep water hoses from being accidentally dragged across planting beds.

The downside of sides is mainly that there doesn't seem to be an ideal material from which to construct them. Most wood rots in constant contact with soil. Naturally rot-resistant wood is usually either expensive or environmentally dubious or, like western cedar, both. Railroad ties and pressure-treated wood, even the newer kinder, gentler ACQ-treated wood are considered too likely to leach undesirable chemicals into your food supply. Cement blocks take up too much space and harbor slugs. There are some environmentally responsible boards made from recycled plastic, but they are pricey.

I have grown crops in beds with several different types of sides, as well as with no sides. My favorite material is untreated wood. It doesn't last forever, but it is easy to work with, non-toxic, and relatively inexpensive. Check around for a lumber mill in your area where outer slabs cut from logs may be had for free. Slabs can give your garden a rustic log-cabin-on-the-prairie look. Untreated wood sides will usually have to be replaced in two to four years, depending mainly on how thick the wood is. Oak and other hardwoods will easily outlast pine. Treating the wood with linseed oil or other natural preservative may extend its useful life somewhat but may not be worth the cost and effort.

Making raised bed sides from two-inch-thick poured concrete slabs will give you pretty much permanent beds, but it is somewhat labor and energy intensive. If you want to build a curved bed, ferro-cement is one of the best choices. Ferro-cement is a thin, durable material made by pressing wet mortar into several layers of wire mesh. Once you get the knack of it, ferro-cement can be formed into whatever shape you like, opening up some Dr. Seuss-inspired garden possibilities.

If you are not short of space and you don't need a super tidy-looking garden, the best option is often to make beds without sides. Not having sides on your beds will eliminate a favorite slug hang out. It also removes the irritation of perennial weeds with roots half in the bed and half in the path. The obvious drawback with no sides is that some of the soil will slide down into the paths. Initially, this is a problem, but gradually a web of soil life begins to hold the beds in shape despite the lure of gravity. Some gardeners use the paths for informal compost making. Putting a thick organic mulch of some kind on the paths raises their level and helps to hold the beds in place. At the end of the growing season, the mulch in the paths can be added to the beds as it is or after further composting. Any soil from the beds that does spill into the path simply enriches that compost.

In areas with sandy, fast-draining soil, there is far less advantage to raised beds. In these conditions, permanent planting beds on ground level will still provide many of the benefits of raised beds without inducing excessive drainage and leaching of nutrients. The ground-level beds will still provide for a better ratio of plants to path, avoid soil compaction, and allow you to focus resources just where the crops are growing. You may want low sides to let you know where the paths end and the beds start and to keep hoses from being dragged over your plants.

Soil Improvement

We all live on a ball that is 8,000 miles in diameter. More than two thirds of its surface is covered with salt water. On the remainder, there is a remarkable skin of soil. A few inches to several feet thick, soil consists of fine rock material, organic matter, water, and air. We get about four percent of all our food from the sea and a tiny percentage from soil-less or hydroponic agriculture. The rest of our food depends on soil being able to support the growth of plants.

Most soil is formed by natural forces breaking down rock. This process of native, or parent, rocks eroding to form soil is continually going on, but the rate of this natural soil formation is extremely slow, especially if you are watching. Hot, humid areas form soil faster that cold, dry regions, but a worldwide average rate of natural soil formation is about one inch every 500 years. When the top inch of our soil started forming, Columbus had just gotten home from finding the New World and Mongols had just breeched the Great Wall of China to overrun the Ming Dynasty. This pokey rate of natural formation makes soil functionally a non-renewable resource.

Clay, silt, and sand are words used to describe the particle size of soil components. Clay is by far the smallest, silt is intermediate, and sand is by far the largest. Sand particles are at least 1,000 times larger than clay particles. There are myriad variations, but typically it goes like this: shale and feldspar break down into clays; granite and limestone into silt; and quartz and sandstone into sand. Older soils tend to have more clay because the rocks are very gradually broken into smaller particles. The proportion of the different-sized particle determines a soil's texture.

If you were to win a hypothetical garden lottery, you would be awarded with an ideal soil in which to grow your vegetable crops. This ideal soil would be made up of roughly equal parts of clay, silt, and sand, creating a soil texture called *loam*. It would be slightly acidic, having pH of about 6.6.[4] In addition to the loamy mixture of clay, silt, and sand, this dream soil would likely contain somewhere between five and ten percent organic matter. All 14 elements essential to plant growth would be present in amounts adequate for good growth. Half of the total volume of the soil would be solids and the other half equal volumes of air and water. There would be at least three feet of this lottery soil before the crops roots hit an impervious layer.

In the real world, this type of soil is exceedingly rare. Most gardeners start with soil that has too much clay or sand, is too acid or alkaline, and may have only one or two percent organic matter. It might be too densely compacted to hold the ideal amount of air or water, or there may be less than a foot before roots run into an impassable layer of hard-packed clay or rock. The most fundamental work of gardening is to incrementally free the garden soil from its real-world shortcomings and move it closer to its potential ideal. This takes time and hard work, but as soon as the soil begins to improve, the gardener is progressively rewarded. The initial investment of hard work in rebuilding your garden's soil saves you work later in controlling pests, weeding, and watering. It also pays dividends of larger harvests of better-quality food.

One of the best ways to begin transforming your garden is to get a soil test done. This will give you sense of how big your job is going to be. Soil tests are often done for free or for a nominal charge by agricultural extension agents or university agriculture departments. These will usually tell you the soil's pH and identify any deficiency or surplus of phosphorus and potassium. It may be worth spending a little more and getting a more complete test done. For example, Logan Labs does an analysis that includes pH, organic matter, calcium, magnesium, potassium, sodium, boron, iron, manganese, copper, zinc, and aluminum. The results are emailed to you within a week, and the cost is $25 as of March 2014 (go to Loganlabs.com for details).

It is difficult to change the basic texture of your soil. Theoretically, you could haul in sand to add to clay soil or bring in clay to mix with sandy soil. However, as most gardeners quickly learn, soil is heavy. The top foot of soil on an average-sized (600 square feet) home garden weighs about 44,000 pounds. That's a lot of wheelbarrow loads. For large gardens or small farms, it is a complete impossibility. The top foot of soil on one acre weighs about 1,600 tons. The environmental impact of digging up and transporting that much sand or clay would be significant, and you would still face the daunting task of mixing the soil components together thoroughly. So, to a large extent, you are stuck with your soil texture: the basic proportions of clay, silt, and sand.

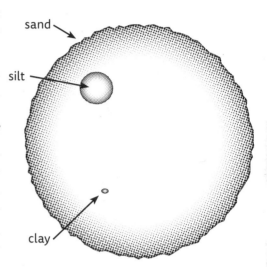

You can, however, make changes in other aspects of your soil that can help compensate for a less-than-ideal texture. The simplest of these changes is to correct the pH. Usually the quickest way to increase the pH of acid soils is to add finely ground agricultural limestone or sifted wood ashes. Wood ashes are more soluble and faster acting but can be more disruptive to soil biology if over applied. Ground limestone is a safer bet, though you should avoid using hydrated or slaked lime. Most soil tests will suggest how much agricultural limestone to apply. Soils that have a pH of 7.5 or higher are considered too alkaline for most plants. Adding sulfur powder is the simplest way to lower the pH.

Both ground limestone and powdered sulfur are best applied in the fall or at end of the crop season so that they have time to become incorporated into the soil before spring crops are set out. If a large pH correction needs to be made, it is a good idea to spread the limestone or sulfur in two different applications at least one month apart. Pine needle and oak leaf mulches will lower soil pH slightly, and manure will often raise pH slightly. Adding compost to your soil has an unusual buffering effect, making acid soils less acid and alkaline soils less alkaline. Like ground limestone and sulfur, compost is also usually best applied in the fall or after crops come out.

While your soil's texture may be very difficult to alter, its structure can certainly be modified in your favor. Structure refers to how the soil particles get along with each other. The volume of a well-structured soil is about one-quarter air and one-quarter water. The open spaces for the air and water are called *pores*. Compacted soil lacks pore space and, as a result, does not have good structure for growing crops. In order to form pores, soil particles need to be loosely clumped together, or *aggregated*. The best way to increase clumping, and therefore pores, is to add organic matter.

Organic matter is basically plants and animals. Ranging from the still living, through the bio-chemically active recently deceased, to the highly stable dead, different types of organic matter perform different services in the soil. A teaspoon of garden soil will contain over a billion live organisms. Most of them are actively eating and breaking down dead plant stems and roots, and in the process, turning them into useful nutrients for new plants. As they chew their way through their food supply of the recently dead plants and animals, soil organisms release organic acids that speed the breakdown of rock particles. They also produce *glomalin* a sticky gelatinous substance that clumps soil particles together and makes pores. *Humus* is the stable dark brown or black remains after all the easily harvested food is removed from organic matter. Humus is especially good at holding water and nutrients.

Organic matter is usually best added to the garden either as compost or by incorporating cover crops. Compost is a way to recycle wastes, making them into a valuable substance that can condition and fertilize your soil. There are several ways to go about it. Probably the best for home gardeners is to make a pile roughly three feet high and three feet on each side by adding alternate layers of carbon-rich material, such as straw or fallen leaves, with thinner layers of nitrogen-rich material such kitchen scraps, manure, or fresh grass clippings. The pile should be moist but not dripping wet.

The advantage of making a pile this large is that it heats up enough to kill most weed seeds and pathogens. Turning the pile twice will mix the outer ingredients into the center exposing them to higher temperatures. The compost is finished when it is black with an earthy smell and you are unable to recognize any of the original ingredients. Finished compost can be applied to the garden beds as is or pushed through a ¼-inch hardware cloth screen to make a more uniform material for starting plants. Anything that won't pass through the screen can be sent back for further composting.

Cover crops, or *green manure crops* as they are sometimes called, are plants grown mainly to improve the soil rather than to provide food. They are especially important anywhere that gardeners don't have access to enough organic matter to make sufficient compost. All cover crops capture carbon

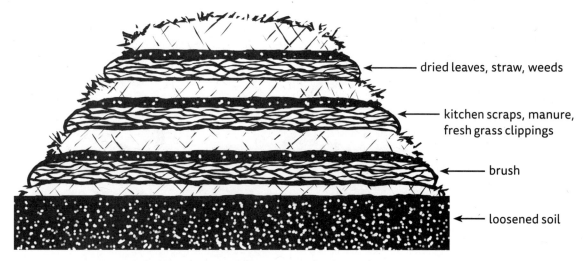

Compost pile (showing content layers)

from the air and convert it to organic matter. Leguminous cover crops, which include peas, beans, clovers, and alfalfa, also capture nitrogen from the air. This nitrogen allows more proteins to be formed, which increases the biomass and ultimately the soil organic matter.

Cover crops can be grown in a separate area and then added to compost piles or brought into the garden to serve as mulch. Cover crops can sometimes be grown in between rows of crops. This is called *intercropping*. Some covers can be grown over the winter, when the garden would otherwise be dormant. Cover crops are most effective when cut just before flowering. They can be chopped and mixed into the top layer of soil or left on top to slowly break down. When the cover crop is mowed and left on top of the soil for two or three weeks, holes can be punched through it to plant seedlings. The slowly decomposing cover crop acts as mulch for the young plants. This technique is becoming more popular because it adds organic matter without disturbing the soil, requires less labor, and results in high yields.

Starting Plants
Start Your Own Leaf Crops

Once you have a spot picked out and have begun improving your soil, it is time to start growing some edible leaf crops. Most familiar annual crops, such as spinach, lettuce, kale, Swiss chard, mustard greens, and turnips

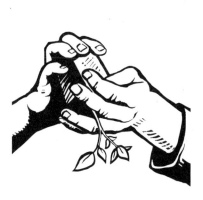

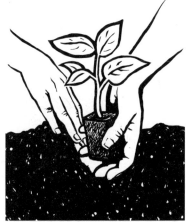

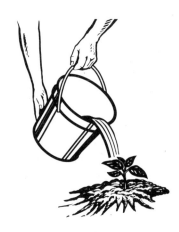

Gently remove transplant from its container.

Place transplant seedling in loosened soil.

Water new transplants thoroughly.

are started from seed. Seed for common varieties can be bought from local stores. Sometimes farm supply stores will measure out small amounts of popular seed varieties from their bulk seed containers. This is usually cheaper than buying seed packets. Seed companies usually offer much greater variety through their Internet stores. But be aware that shipping and handling charges can bump up the cost of small orders.

You can sow seeds directly in the garden beds or start seeds in potting soil in small cups or trays and transplant the young plants into the garden after two to five weeks. Plant seed about twice as deep as the seed is long. Planting too deep is the most common cause of vegetable seed not germinating. Seeds that are old or especially hard will germinate better if they are soaked for a few hours in warm water before planting. Because plants are the most vulnerable during germination and early growth, it often pays to start seeds in potting soil, with some extra care and protection from the elements. Less seed is wasted when plants are started in this way, and it is much easier to establish the optimal distances between plants when they go into the beds.

Seeds are one of the biggest expenses facing gardeners, though it is sometimes possible to get seeds for free. Seed libraries are gradually being established throughout the country. These are like book libraries, sometimes even run through the public libraries, except that they loan garden seeds instead of books. The agreement is that if the plants do well, you allow some of them to develop mature seeds and return a portion of those to the library for other patrons to borrow for the next season. A good place to check for seed libraries near you is richmondgrowsseeds.org.

Once you gain a little experience gardening, you can begin saving some seed from your own plants. Save seeds from healthy open pollinated or non-hybrid plants. (Hybrid plants are created by crossing two different varieties. They are normally labeled as "hybrid" on the seed packet—and they are usually more expensive. Hybrid seeds tend to grow well, but saving their seed is not a good option for home gardeners. Many hybrids are sterile, and those that aren't rarely reproduce the desired traits.) Seeds should be mature and dry before they are harvested. They will keep best if they stay cool and dry. Usually, late afternoon on a sunny day is the best time to harvest seeds.

Volunteers

We usually think of volunteers as civic-minded folks who work without pay taking meals to old people, cataloging library books, or cleaning up our roadsides. On bad days, they may be filling sandbags or fighting forest fires. In the garden, a volunteer is a useful plant that no one planted. It volunteers to grow where it will, usually from seed dropped from last year's plants.

Some leaf crops drop seed abundantly and regularly produce volunteers. Almost without fail, I get plenty of free sets from vine spinach (*Basella rubra*), quail grass (*Celosia argentea*), red Hopi amaranth, (*Amaranthus cruentus*), spider wisp (*Cleome gynandra*), purslane (*Portulaca oleracae*), orach (*Atriplex hortensis*), shiso (*Perilla frutescens*), rice beans (*Vigna umbellata*), hyacinth beans (*Lablab purpureus*), dill, and others every spring.

In addition to avoiding the cost of buying new seed, the volunteers have a couple of advantages over planted seeds. They wait until the soil temperature is adequate before sprouting. Volunteers have also gone through at least one round of local selection. That is, they are the offspring of plants that grew well enough to bear viable seed in the actual conditions of your garden.

Because volunteers often sprout in profusion, the most vigorous individuals can be selected and transplanted to desirable spacing. The others, I let grow until they begin to interfere with other plantings, then I cut the leafy tops and either eat them or dry them for later use. Some of them—notably vine spinach, amaranth, and quail grass—can be harvested in this way two or three times, providing a good supply of high-quality organic greens with no cost or effort other than the harvest. When they begin crowding other crops, I slice them off at the ground level with a very sharp hoe. It doesn't seem fair, but unfortunately not all the volunteers can be allowed to reach maturity and have families of their own.

Some leaf crops are better propagated vegetatively from stem cuttings (discussed shortly). Among these are: chaya, grapes, katuk, Okinawa spinach, sweet potatoes, wolfberry, and many perennial herbs, such as rosemary and mints. Some plants, such as moringa and vine spinach can be propagated by *either* seed or stem cuttings. When you have the choice, starting from seed usually makes stronger plants, but they may take a bit longer to get established.

Usually, the best stem cuttings are about eight inches long and taken from one- or two-year-old growth. Some plants, such as chaya, moringa, and katuk may not have any leaves on the stem section you use. Others such as sweet potatoes, vine spinach, and wolfberry will. Strip the leaves from the bottom half of the cut stem. Push the stem about one-third of its length into good soil. Make sure the same end is up when you plant the stem. You may want to mark it in some way. Keep stem cuttings moist but not wet until new growth appears. Stems can be planted directly into the garden, but often do better if they are started in a container and transplanted to the garden after they develop some roots. Stem cuttings are frequently free for the asking because gardeners typically prune their perennial leaf crops at least once a year and may be happy to share the trimmed stems with fellow growers.

Root division is another way to propagate plants. This is done by breaking up the tightly packed roots into smaller clumps and planting those clumps separately. Comfrey, asparagus, and daylilies are examples of plants propa-

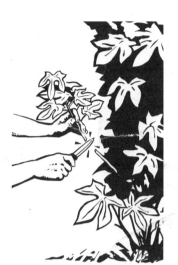 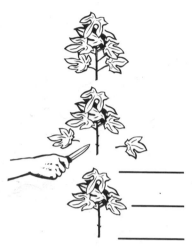 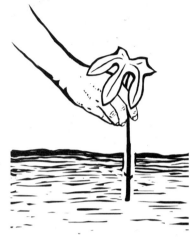

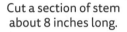

| Cut a section of stem about 8 inches long. | Remove at least half the leaves. | Push the stem cutting ⅓ of its length into wet soil. |

…d by root division. Among leaf crops, garlic chives (*Allium tuberosum*) falls into this category.

Water

Water is a colorless, odorless, tasteless, transparent liquid. It can also be solid (as ice) or a gas (as vapor, or steam). It covers about 70 percent of the earth's surface. Water is the universal solvent. It is the vehicle for transferring the substances that make up the physical basis of life from one place to another. Water is constantly moving. Clouds roll by. Rain pours down. Rivers run to the sea. Water is easy to misplace, but hard to really lose.

The water from our urine or from flooded suburban basements drifts up to the sky as vapor, the same as with the water in clear mountain streams. When that water vapor condenses, it falls from the clouds on everything. It is the ultimate recyclable resource.

We use more water for growing food than for any other human activity. About half of all the farms and gardens in the world are in areas with frequent water shortages. Lack of water is one of the main causes of poverty. So, using it efficiently is important. One of the most important tasks facing a gardener is to make sure that plants have an adequate supply of water. Plants that have enough water, especially when they are young, are healthier and produce more food than water-stressed plants.

Most leaf crops are over 80 percent water. They usually need about an inch of rain per week. More may be needed when it is hot and dry and less when it is cool and cloudy. You can compensate for rainfall shortages by watering deeply once a week. Young plants with shallow roots may benefit from more frequent watering, but shallow irrigation doesn't encourage the growth of strong deep roots in older plants.

Beginning gardeners often underestimate how much water their plants need. It may pay to do a bit of math. An inch of water over a typical 4 by 25 foot bed is about 62 gallons, or 520 pounds (important to know if you are hauling it in buckets). An average home garden of 600 square feet will have about 400 square feet of garden beds and require roughly 250 gallons of water a week. Over a ten-week stretch with no rain, this adds up to a requirement of 2,500 gallons of water.

Most locations won't have ten weeks without a significant rain, but figuring it this way provides a bit of margin for a dry summer.

So, where do we get this water? Many gardeners are turning away from using chlorinated drinking-quality water to irrigate their gardens. The chlorine poses little problem to the plants, but the environmental impact of treating and pumping the water is significant. Catching some of the water that falls on roofs is an obvious idea. The use of plastic 55-gallon rain barrels to supplement garden water supply has become popular recently, and it may be a step in the right direction. However, a full barrel holds less than what one bed needs for a week.

Much larger containers would be needed to capture enough to make a real difference. A lot of water falls on roofs. A 2,000-square-foot house with a typical overhang in a one-inch rain will intercept 1,400 gallons of distilled water on its way back to the ocean. A thousand gallon rainwater harvesting tank with screens, overflow and hose connections can be bought for about $600–800.[5] It can fit nicely under a gutter and can gravity feed water to your garden beds. A small pond is another possibility for catching relevant quantities of water for your garden.

The very best place to store water for leaf crops is often in the soil itself. Increasing the organic matter and the depth of topsoil will enable your garden soil to capture and hold much more water from a rain and allow you to water less often. Assuming an average clay content, a 100-square-foot garden bed that is seven percent organic matter can hold about 315 gallons of water. The same-sized bed that has only two percent organic matter can hold only about 158 gallons of water. This can be the difference between a good food crop and failure.

Plants need water for photosynthesis, for transpiration, for transporting nutrients, for keeping cool, and for several other functions. On an equal weight basis, a healthy garden plant needs about 20 times more water per day than a person. We can reduce the water needs of our crops by slowing down the rate of evaporation—the return of the water to the sky as water vapor. Watering in the early evening is usually best because less water evaporates than when crops are watered in the hot midday sun. Evaporation can also be minimized by root zone irrigation. This is simply putting water below the surface—where the crops' roots are—rather than on the soil surface when hot sun will quickly evaporate it.

This can be done by sinking a clay pot or bucket (with holes in the bottom) in the garden bed. When these are filled, the water seeps slowly into the

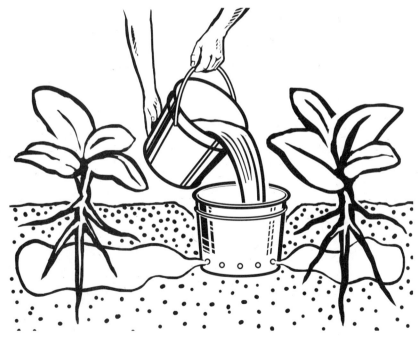

A bucket with holes in the bottom lets water reach
the roots of plants with less loss to evaporation.

ground close to the plant roots. Another simple root zone irrigation technique uses capillary action moving water through a wick made of discarded cloth of some sort. This system works especially well with shallow-rooted plants that require a steady supply of water. A blanket or other similar cloth is laid in a trench 6–10 inches deep then covered with garden soil. Plants are spaced above or just to the side of the wick. One end of the wick cloth stays in a bucket of water that is sunken so that just an inch or two remains above the ground level. As the root zone dries out, water is wicked to it along the buried cloth, providing a steady supply of water to the plant roots while minimizing evaporation losses. If you adopt this method, bear in mind that synthetic materials will last much longer than natural fiber cloth.

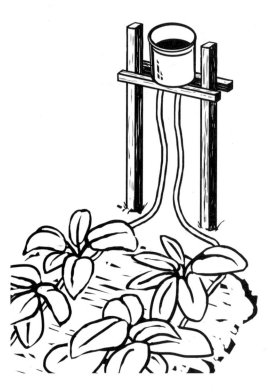

Simple drip irrigation

Another excellent water-conserving technique is the use of drip or soaker hoses. Drip hoses can be placed under or directly on top of the soil. They are typically ¼-inch tubes with tiny holes to release water to your plants. Soaker hoses are similar except that they allow the water to slowly seep through the entire porous hose instead of just the holes. You can try this system on a very small scale by attaching the drip or soaker hose to a raised five-gallon bucket, and letting the plants be watered by gravity. Any drip system needs to use water that contains very little sediment or it will quickly clog.

Whatever method you use to supply water to your garden, it will work better if you place mulch around plants to hold moisture in. Mulch is a protective layer, usually of organic matter, that slows down evaporation. It also keeps soil temperature steady and reduces weeds. Compost, shredded leaves, straw, newspaper, cardboard, and grass clippings (from places where no herbicides have been used) all make good organic mulches.

In regions that have a long dry season, as is the case with much of the tropics, perennial leaf crops will often outperform annual crops. Perennial plants have deeper roots that are more able to reach an underground water source in the dry season.

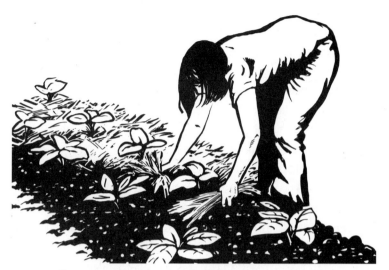

Put straw or other organic material around plants
to prevent weeds and conserve soil moisture.

The Competition: Weeds and Bugs

Shortly after you begin growing vegetables, you will be introduced to the competition: weeds and bugs. Weeds will sip on your crops' sunshine and snack on the improved soil you lovingly prepared. And then there are pests—voracious insects who will feast on the very vegetables you had planned on eating.

Weeds

Weeds are plants growing where you don't want them to grow. They are unwanted guests that compete with your garden plants for sunlight, water, and soil nutrients. Many garden weeds are pioneer plants. These are plants whose ecological role is to quickly reestablish a cover on soil disturbed by flood or fire. They are opportunistic plants that grow quickly and produce a large quantity of seed in a short time. After a flood or a fire, these are the first plants to grow on the disturbed land. Many weeds, such as lambsquarters and pigweed can barely survive in well-established ecosystems like forests or prairies. They require the advantages that bare disturbed ground provide them. They have become *anthropophilic* species, or species whose population thrives in the presence of humans. Humans gardening and farming create far more disturbed land than do natural events. Minimizing soil disturbance creates fewer opportunities for weeds. No-till agriculture, leaving mowed cover crops on top of the soil, and mulching garden beds significantly reduces soil disturbances and thus opportunities for these weeds.

Controlling weeds is usually the most time consuming and often the least pleasant part of gardening. "Too many weeds" is the most common reason given when people decide to stop growing vegetables. It is nearly impossible to completely avoid weeds, but there are a few relatively simple steps that can shrink the problem to a manageable level.

The first principle is to provide weeds with as little disturbed bare soil as possible. Cover bare ground with organic mulch or plant cover crops so that soil is not available for weed seeds to germinate in. The second basic element of weed control is to kill annual weeds before they can produce seeds. Some weeds, such as pigweed, can produce 100,000 viable seeds each year. Some of these seeds can lie dormant in the soil for several years. Experienced gardeners warn: "One year to seed, nine years to weed."

Cut weeds when they are young and tender. This can be done very quickly. It is easier to go through the garden several times, cutting tender young weeds just below the soil surface than to wait until they are bigger and have stronger roots. It takes little effort using a sweeping motion with a long-handled, razor-sharp collinear-type hoe. Slicing with a collinear-type hoe puts less strain on the back muscles than chopping weeds with a heavier traditional hoe. It is basically just a sharp blade on a long lightweight stick. It is held with thumbs pointing up and used like a broom in an upright stance. As with any hoe, it works much better if the blade is frequently sharpened with a file. Collinear hoes are not widely available yet, but can be bought online through garden supply stores. Variations on these handy tools could be easily made by a local metal worker as a cottage industry.

Perennial weeds, such as Johnson grass (*Sorghum halepense*) or yellow nutsedge (*Cyperus esculentus*), can be more difficult to get rid of than annual weeds. Because they can reproduce through underground rhizomes, it can seem like a futile exercise chopping them down only to have them pop up again. Gardeners often surrender prematurely. The reality is that the underground portion of the plants is completely

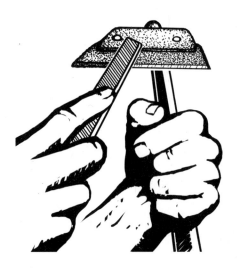

Sharpening hoe
for easier weed control.

dependent on its above-ground counterpart to photosynthesize and supply energy. If you *continue* clipping off the tops, eventually the underground rhizomes with run out of energy and die off.

Sometimes perennial weeds can be smothered by a dense planting of a more desirable cover crop. Velvet beans (*Mucuna pruriens*), buckwheat, Sudan-grass, and vetch are sometimes planted for this purpose. Closely planted indeterminate-type cowpeas, hyacinth beans (*Lablab purpureus*) and sweet potatoes can also be used. They have the advantage of having edible, nutritious leaves that can be partially harvested.

Especially stubborn perennial weeds can be killed by covering the soil with a clear plastic sheet for four to six weeks during a hot time of year. This can raise the soil temperature enough to kill most perennial weed·roots, most weed seeds, and many harmful nematodes and fungi. The plastic needs to be well sealed over moist soil for the best results. You will not be able to grow crops while killing the weeds with this method.

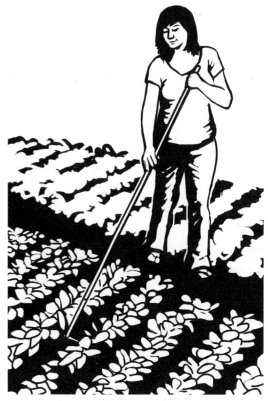

Less back strain standing up straight with collinear hoe.

Eat Your Weedies

Remember that many weeds have edible leaves. Often, they are more nutritious than the vegetable crops that they threaten. As you learn to harvest and eat them, they stop being weeds. They are tastiest and most nutritious when eaten before they flower and produce seed. They can be harvested either by cutting them off at the ground or by uprooting them. The following are among the common garden weeds that are edible and nutritious:

- Dandelion (*Taraxacum officiale*)
- Lambsquarters (*Chenopodium album*)
- Pigweed (*Amaranthus retroflexus*)
- Purslane (*Portulaca oleracea*)

- Dock (*Rumex crispus*)
- Chickweed (*Stellaria media*)
- Plantain (*Plantago major*)
- Stinging nettles (*Urtica dioica*)

Pests

About one-fourth of the world's entire food crop is lost to insects and plant disease. That is a lot of potential food to lose. Deer, groundhogs, rabbits, mice, turtles, birds, and tens of thousands of species of insects are interested in eating what you are growing. Food lost to pests becomes a lot less abstract when you are growing food for your table in a kitchen garden. You can see the insects eating your food—and often making a mess in the process. The messy eating habits of many pests leave your crops with open wounds that foster plant diseases and even greater losses.

Larger pests can often be dealt with best by fencing in your garden or by introducing predators. There are plenty of fencing products available at farm supply stores, and likely, you can get some advice on what type of fence will best deter what types of pests. Deer, of course, need the tallest fence, as they are excellent jumpers. If their population is exceeding their normal food supply, they will take chances to jump into your garden. Groundhogs, on the other hand, will burrow under most fences unless they extend at least a foot below ground. Ammonia and soap, or olive oil-soaked rags in groundhogs holes will often encourage them to relocate. Diluted hot pepper sauce sprayed on the leaves of your garden plants may discourage many mammals from feeding. Spraying must be repeated after rains. And don't forget your pets. Cats and dogs will threaten, if not kill and eat, many of the herbivores that are inclined to eat our gardens.

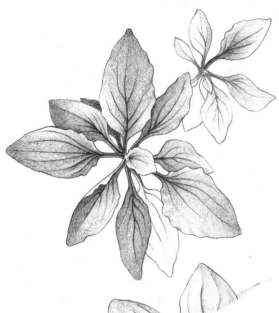

Plantain,
Plantago major

Paradoxically, it is usually the smaller pests that create the larger problems. Microscopic beings that damage crops including some bacteria, fungi, and viruses are usually considered diseases rather than pests. Diseases caused by these pests are almost invariably easier to prevent than to cure.

A few tips for avoiding plant disease in your garden:
• Don't plant moldy seed.
• Remove any diseased plants from your garden and don't use them to

make compost. The heat of the compost pile is not always high enough
to kill mold spores and viruses.

- Wash the inside of plant containers at the end of a growing season if
you plan to reuse the container.
- Space plants far enough apart to allow for air movement. This is especially important in humid climates or in low spots.
- Change where you plant your crops within your garden so that members of the same plant family don't follow each other.
- Use compost as a protective mulch around plants. Generous use of
finished compost can reduce virus and fungus problems.
- Try spraying any crops that show signs of fungal or virus disease with a
tea made from nettle leaf, horsetail, or compost.

The Problem with Poison

Insecticides are poisons that kill insects. Herbicides
are poisons that kill plants. Starting in earnest after
the Second World War, the chemical industry began
producing and promoting ever-greater quantities of these poisons.
The concept has been basically to identify the enemy's weakness and
kill it as cheaply and profitably as possible. The appeal of using pesticides to grow food is straightforward. It takes less effort to spray a crop
with insecticides and herbicides than to pick off insect and hoe weeds.
Let's use Mexican bean beetles, a common garden and farm pest as an
example, although the basic principle holds with most other pests. Assume Mexican bean beetles are ruining $100 worth of your bean crop
and you can kill them with $10 worth of insecticide; you save $90.

So far so good. But we haven't gotten very far. Poisons are not good
to eat. It is not always obvious when a substance introduced into our
environment is causing health problems. The worst offenders have
been banned, but no one wants to eat pesticide residues. Children, because they are creating new cells so quickly, are especially vulnerable
to potential problems from pesticide residues.

In addition to problems tied to direct human consumption of
residues, there is some collateral damage. Innocent bystanders such

as birds, fish, and frogs are often victims of the poisons because they accumulate in their systems. Insecticide use can also cause secondary or rebound infestations. There are 17 known predators of bean beetles that offer some biological control. If an insecticide is more effective on those predator populations than on the target beetles, the Mexican bean beetles may return in greater numbers because of the lack of predators. Sometimes the rebound or secondary infestation is with another species. Suppose, in addition to bean beetles, aphids are eating my beans, but the aphid population is being controlled by ladybugs. The insecticide kills the bean beetles but also the ladybugs. Without the ladybug predation, the aphid population quickly builds— and now I am looking for an insecticide to spray on *them*.

The biggest problem with the routine use of poisons in agriculture, however, is far more elemental. It is programmed into the heart of evolutionary biology. A species that quickly produces large numbers of offspring (and virtually all insect and weed pest species are in this category) will quickly develop genetic resistance to a given poison.

Any trait in any naturally occurring population can be plotted along a bell-shaped curve. Here, the trait is resistance to a pesticide, and the population is the Mexican bean beetles in my bean field. The figure opposite shows the bean beetle population after the first year of spraying an insecticide. The beetles to the left side of the curve are the least resistant. Most of the beetles have average resistance and are therefore in the middle, or the hump, of the curve. On the left side of the curve are the beetles with the greatest resistance to the pesticide.

The poison is very potent and kills *all* the beetles with low or average resistance. Ninety percent of the most resistant beetles are also killed. Let's say there were 10,000 bean beetles on my plants before I sprayed, and the pesticide killed 9,900 or 99 percent of them. I have protected my bean crop but at the same time I have made sure that only those beetles with the highest level of genetic resistance to the pesticide will be able to reproduce and pass on their resistance genes.

Insecticides have been widely used since about 1950. Since then, about three generations of humans have been exposed to these

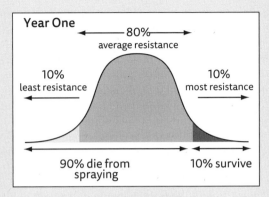

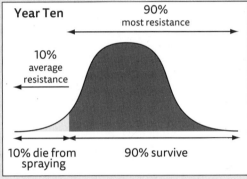

Mexican bean beetle natural selection
for pesticide resistance.

chemicals in the environment. However, Mexican bean beetles have
two to three generations *per season*. Females can lay up to 500 eggs at
a time. So, beetles spawn 180 generations in the same time we generate three—giving the beetles lots of chances to genetically adapt
to the pesticide. The combination of multiple annual generations,
large numbers of offspring (some insects have 30,000 offspring),
and extreme environmental pressure from the fatal spray creates an
evolutionary incubator. Within 60 years of use, at least 500 species of
insects have developed significant genetic resistance to an insecticide
that was once effective against them.

A parallel development has been the increasing genetic resistance to herbicides in weed populations. At least six weeds, including ragweed and pigweed, have already developed some degree of genetic resistance to glyphosate, the key ingredient in Monsanto's Round Up herbicide. With herbicides, we are trying to rein in a lot of adaptive power. Each pigweed (*Amaranthus retroflexus*) plant for example, can generate tens of thousands of seeds. The seeds can germinate and grow so quickly that the plant can produce several generations each season. The number of distinct genetic possibilities over ten years greatly exceeds the space on my calculator. This is not an abstract mathematical problem. By the summer of 2009, herbicide-resistant Palmer amaranth was already making cotton harvest nearly impossible and threatening soybean fields in the southeastern US.

Genetic resistance is how evolution responds to the widespread use of poison. An even more accelerated example of this type of natural selection has occurred with genetic resistance to antibiotics in bacteria. For instance, it is now assumed that most staphylococcus bacteria in the United States have synthesized penicillinase, an enzyme that neutralizes penicillin, rendering that antibiotic nearly useless against staphylococcus infections. The offspring of insects and weeds seem like the products of long, thoughtful courtships compared to the geometry of bacterial reproduction. This is why we need to continually create new antibiotics and why the US Centers for Disease Control says "antibiotic resistance is one of the world's most pressing public health threats."

Insect pests can take a lot of the fun—and food—out of gardening, and people have spent a long time thinking about how to deal with them. After 10,000 years of agriculture, what we have figured out is that the best way to manage insect pests is to keep them guessing. Best to bring a whole toolbox full of strategies and mix them up. Insects can evolve resistance to a poison because poison is a simple, one-dimensional strategy. They can't simultaneously develop resistance to a more complex mixture of disincentives.

Sometimes called Integrated Pest Management (IPM), the whole-toolbox scheme of mixed strategies is intended to keep pest damage at a tolerable level, while minimizing incidental harm to other parts of the ecosystem. It begins with careful observation. You need to find out what is eating your plants before the damage is too great to reverse. Use a magnifying glass if necessary. Several online databases can help you to identify insect pests visually. Most states have home garden IPM information available for free through agricultural extension offices. A good introduction to garden-scale IPM is an online slide show from the University of Florida at sarasota.ifas .ufl.edu.

The integrated approach requires you to accept some losses and some visual damage from pests. You can't get—and you shouldn't expect—complete control of insect pests. When you determine that the damage from an insect is approaching your limit, begin implementing progressively stronger measures until you have adequate control.

Some IPM measures are given below, roughly from least intrusive to more intrusive. Of course, you may want to take several of these actions simultaneously.

- Keep improving your garden soil. Healthy plants growing in healthy soil have fewer insect problems.
- Grow crops that are not prone to damage from a particular insect. For example, my yardlong beans are little bothered by the same bean beetles that decimate ordinary kidney beans. Extension agents and seasoned local gardeners are good resources for this kind of information, but ultimately your own experience is the most important.
- Grow a complex mixture of plants, including fragrant herbs and flowers. This confuses insects' ability to locate their target plants.
- Use scarecrows, rubber snakes and owls, spinning pinwheels, aluminum foil strips, or other tricky devices to frighten and confuse pests.
- Time your planting schedule to avoid periods of peak insect activity.
- Attract birds, lizards, frogs, turtles, bats, and toads that eat harmful insects. Small ponds, birdhouses and perches, and overturned clay pots acting as "toad houses" make your garden attractive to these insect-eating animals.
- Plant trap crops. For example, rabbits will prefer eating a trap crop of clover to your bean crop. Groundhogs prefer alfalfa to sweet potatoes.
- Use physical barriers such as fence, screen, mesh, or fabric row covers to keep pests out. Row covers can be especially helpful for plants that need protection from insects only when they are young and tender.

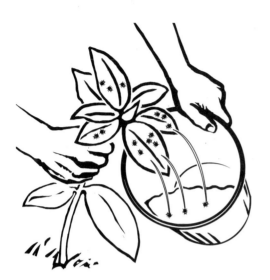

Shake beetles off into bucket of water.

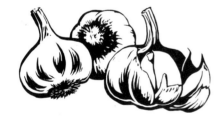

- Handpick insects. Early morning is when most insects are the slowest and easiest to pick. Many insects will drop from leaves if they are lightly shaken. Hold a bucket with a small amount of water in it below where you shake. If you or your neighbor has chickens, feed the insects to chickens. They are very high in the protein and other nutrients that improve egg production.
- Make repellents by soaking any combination of the following in water for 24 hours: garlic, marigolds, chili peppers, tobacco, mint, or tansy. Strain and spray on affected crops.
- Only if you are unable to gain control using these safe measure should you consider using insecticides. Try natural insecticides such as spinosad, neem, Bt, or pyrethrums. (Clemson University has an excellent webpage on how to choose low-toxicity insecticides at clemson.edu.) Wait at least a week after spraying to harvest the crop. Wash food well before eating after using any repellents or natural insecticides. It is usually better to plant a bit more to make up for moderate insect damage than to expose your family to agricultural poisons in their food.

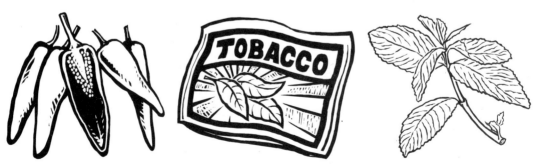

Ingredients for repellent (above left to right: garlic, chili pepper, tobacco, mint)

Functional Biophilia: Organic vs. Conventional Agriculture

Roughly four percent of our food is considered to be *organically* grown, with the remaining 96 percent *conventionally* grown. What do these terms mean?

Conventional agriculture really just describes whatever techniques are popular for commercial growing at any given time. At this time, conventional agriculture is focused on the use of crops that have been genetically modified to withstand heavy herbicide application. Fertility is provided mainly through the application of potent soluble fertilizers, and most tasks are mechanized. If organic agriculture were more popular, it would be conventional.

In the US, "organic" has increasingly become a legal term that means a product conforms to the standards of the National Organic Program and is thus allowed to use their organic logo. Those standards stress the avoidance of most synthetic fertilizers, herbicides, and pesticides, as well as sewage sludge, genetically modified crops, and the routine use of growth hormones and antibiotics. The standards emphasize maintaining soil health with compost, cover crops, manures, animal by-products, seaweeds, and naturally occurring minerals.

Life, as we have come to know it, relies on the presence of large molecules built around chains of carbon atoms. In chemistry, simply containing carbon atoms is enough to make something organic. In common usage, "organic" means relating to organisms or living beings. People sometime ask, "Do you garden organically?" I might answer that I am trying to develop a more organic world view.

It is a big shift in how we see things, and big shifts don't come fast and easy. In 1543, about the time our most recent inch of topsoil began forming, Nicolaus Copernicus published his treatise *On the Revolutions of the Heavenly Spheres* which proposed that the Earth revolved around the Sun, rather than the other way around. Though the evidence was convincing, it took about 200 years for that idea to catch on. Space travel was still a ways off, so why was there so much resistance to the idea?

It wasn't the change in the status of the Earth and Sun that was so upsetting as much as the implications about the centrality of humans. Our home planet was starting to look like a smaller player in a bigger universe. Religion and culture have long assured us that we are special creatures living in a unique place, and science has repeatedly tempered that assurance with perspective gained by carefully observing other creatures and other places.

Today, science is showing us that our world is enormously more alive, or, if you will, more organic, than we had ever suspected. This new information is forcing us to reconsider the primacy of human experience in the grand scheme of things. We may resist the idea for 200 years, but the evidence is building daily that our existence depends on the health of thousands of species of largely microscopic living beings.

What we only recently came to recognize as tiny germs that could infect us if they weren't killed, are now looking more like citizens of biotic communities whose complex patterns of interactions provide us with many benefits, as well as the better-known dangers. The human body, it turns out, is home to over 100 trillion bacteria, outnumbering our human cells roughly ten to one.[6] The bacteria actually protect us against many infections by controlling the acidity of our guts, strengthening the tissue lining our digestive tract, and increasing our disease-fighting white blood cells. They allow us to more fully digest our food and synthesize several essential vitamins.

Our war on germs seems to be sliding toward constructive engagement. Even the medical establishment that had been leading the charge appears to be calling for a truce, suggesting that we curtail our enthusiasm for anti-bacterial sponges, soaps, wipes, rinses, and sprays because they may be unintentionally breeding antibiotic-resistant pathogens.

Everywhere we look (assuming we are willing to look through a microscope) we are finding life in mind-blowing numbers and variety. Our skin, our teeth, our guts are home to densely populated multicultural communities of small organisms. Every breath we suck into our lungs is alive with creatures too tiny to see or to feel. Beyond the boundaries of our bodies, the raw passion of these tiny beings to adapt and survive inspires confidence in the force of life. The most amazing are the *extremophiles* who settle in the dangerous neighborhoods like the inside of rocks under mile-deep water or in volcanic vents hot enough to instantly boil water.

If you are ready to embrace life in its fullness, you are developing an organic world view. A good place to wallow in life is the soil in your garden. The organic world has its headquarters in the soil. The Earth's wafer-thin covering of soil contains roughly three times as much carbon as the ten-mile-thick blanket of air. Soil also holds about four times as much carbon as all of the life above the soil. The table below gives a glimpse of the range of life below your lettuce plants.

It is in the care and feeding of these soil food webs that the "organic" and "conventional" approaches to growing food most differ. Conventional agriculture is predicated on the belief that plants can't tell the difference between nutrients supplied as soluble synthetic fertilizers and nutrients that arrive at the plants' roots from the complex interactions of soil organisms. This premise is based on the outdated concept that plants are basically stupid and passive.

Conventional agriculture has long required overlooking the sophisticated relationships among plants and soil organisms. One such association is between plant roots and mycorrhizal fungi. Some of these fungi, called arbuscular mycorrhiza actually live within plant root cells, while others attach themselves to the outer surface of the roots. Plants provide the fungi with sugars formed in their leaves and in exchange the fungi offer the plant better access to

Table 2. Life in One Acre of Healthy Garden Soil

Mammals	2 lb
Protozoa	133 lb
Earthworms	900 lb
Insects	900 lb
Algae	900 lb
Bacteria	2000 lb
Fungi	2400 lb

Note: Chart information comes from Lowenfels, Jeff, and Wayne Lewis. *Teaming with Microbes: The Organic Gardener's Guide to the Soil Food Web*. Portland, Oregon: Timber Press, 2010. page 28

water and nutrients, especially phosphorus. Appearing in plant fossils from 400 million years ago, these mycorrhizal cooperative arrangements exist in about 80 percent of modern plant species studied.

Perhaps even better known is the partnership of leguminous (bean and pea family) plants and rhizobia bacteria. The plants provide sugars made in their leaves to feed the bacteria and in exchange the bacteria provide nitrogen to the plant. All plants need nitrogen to create proteins, but they can't make use of the element until it has been converted to a nitrate or ammonia form. Rhizobia use the enzyme nitrogenase to convert the nitrogen. Humans can convert it through the industrial process that produces nitrogen fertilizer. The difference is that leguminous plants and their rhizobia bacteria cohorts can convert nitrogen in the air to a usable form for plants at temperatures between 50–90°F (10–32°C). Our industrial process, on the other hand, requires temperatures around 930°F (500°C) and 200 times atmospheric pressure for accomplishing the same thing. So who's stupid?

The term "biophilia" was popularized by a book of the same name by Edward O. Wilson in 1984. It refers to an instinctive "love of life or living systems" that we all share. The biophilia hypothesis helps explain why we think baby animals are cute and why we seek out parks and wince at the sight of bulldozers scraping the vegetation from land. The organic gardener has the capacity to exercise *functional biophilia* by creating conditions that actually increase the amount of life on Earth.

Relatively simple practices such as keeping the ground covered, planting diverse species, recycling wastes into the soil, and growing cover crops, increases soil organic matter and fertility. The richer soil provides stronger plant cover that photosynthesizes better, turning more carbon from the air into living tissue. Rain is absorbed faster and held longer by the improved soil fostering greater life underfoot. If employed over a large enough area, these practices would reverse the damage to global climate systems caused by burning fossil fuels.

Gardeners work with very small plots of land, so their beneficial impact is modest, but it's real. As more people plant gardens and more gardeners learn good organic practices, this benefit will increase. Beyond the increased life in the millions of pea patches, healthy gardens are an important reminder and a powerful symbol of our relationship with life. It is hard to care for what we don't love and hard to love what we don't know. Gardens help us get to know life.

So if someone should ask, "Do you garden organically?" I answer enthusiastically.

7

Stellar Additions

❊ ❊ ❊

Dynamic New Leaf Crops for the Home Garden

A large survey done by the US National Gardening Association in 2009 listed the ten most popular home grown vegetables in this order:

1. Tomatoes
2. Cucumbers
3. Sweet Peppers
4. Beans
5. Carrots
6. Summer Squash
7. Onions
8. Hot Peppers
9. Lettuce
10. Peas

Everything on this list your grandma would have recognized and may have even grown. So, it seems most home gardeners are still pretty conservative in choosing which vegetable plants to grow. This isn't too surprising. People grow what they like to eat, and generally they like to eat what they are used to eating. Growing a few reliable favorites flattens the learning curve and simplifies finding seed and other tasks associated with growing food.

So, why expand the palette if you are happy with the painting? Why not? From amongst the ten most popular home grown vegetables in the US, only some varieties of summer squash are native to the land. If our gardening forefathers (or, quite likely, our foremothers) had been satisfied with what they were already growing, Italians would have no tomatoes for marinara sauce, Indians would have no chilis to fire up their vinadaloo, and Louisiana shrimp gumbo would have to limp along without the okra. These three staple vegetable crops began as stellar additions to earlier gardens.

New crops bring not just dynamic new culinary opportunities but nutritional insurance and greater food security. My Irish ancestors could have used a few productive new crops to go with their potatoes. With shifting global climate patterns, change is literally in the air. Gardeners need a larger botanical toolkit to prepare for the possibility of more severe and less predictable weather and the influx of exotic pests that it may bring.

The mandate of commercial agriculture is too narrowly focused on market solutions to allow for the sort of experimentation that is needed. The drive for volume production and ever-lower labor costs has become a monotonous tribute to financial risk avoidance. Whenever good nutrition and sound ecological management diverge from short-term financial gain, finance rules the day. Some of the resulting nutritional and ecological problems are now literally bred into the very seeds of commercial agriculture.

Gardens are a logical place to begin to flush diversity through our food system. For a growing number of younger gardeners, curiosity and adventure are drawing them toward new crops, new techniques, and new ways of eating what the garden produces. Younger gardeners have likely traveled more than their parents and grandparents and are more familiar with ethnic foods. The latest cohort of vegetable gardeners has also grown up with a greater awareness of environmental issues and are more likely to incorporate ecological perspectives into their food-growing efforts. For many folks new to gardening, increasing the biodiversity of their gardens to improve the efficiency and stability of the system is not an alien idea.

For the adventurous gardener of any age, this chapter offers up a few relatively unfamiliar leaf crops that merit a try. No one wants to eat just greens, so ideally these leafy additions to the garden will complement, not replace, old garden favorites.

In total, there are 21 plants I would like to encourage people to grow for their edible greens. Of the 21, five are discussed as multi-use plants in Chapter 8. They are stellar additions to the garden because they produce tasty, nutritious leaves in addition to healthy grains, flowers, teas, tubers, or berries. These are:

- Grain Amaranth
- Quail Grass
- Roselle
- Sweet Potatoes
- Wolfberry

Another five of the 21 plants are edible cover crops, described in Chapter 11. The plants in this group qualify as stellar additions to your garden because they produce plenty of greens full of vitamins, minerals, and antioxidants, while simultaneously improving the structure and fertility of your soil. These are:

- Alfalfa
- Austrian Winter Peas
- Barley
- Cowpeas
- Wheat

The remaining 11 leaf crops that I recommend for your consideration are covered in this chapter. There are over 1,000 species of plants with edible leaves, so I clearly couldn't include them all. The 11 stellar leaf crops I describe in this chapter have unique attributes that make them likely to be successful additions to the adventurous North American home garden. They are all underutilized as garden plants, and all have nutritious leaves. I hope you will find a few you'd like to try. I think you'll find they are fun to grow and can enhance the value of your home garden.

Chaya, Tree Spinach
(Cnidoscolus aconitifolius, C. chayamansa)

Chaya is an attractive perennial shrub native to the Yucatan peninsula of Mexico and the drier parts of Central America. It is a member of the Euphorbia family, which also includes cassava and poinsettia. The wild forms of chaya can have irritating hairs, or trichomes, on their leaves, but these disappear with cooking. Most domesticated varieties don't have these hairs.

Chaya is a tropical perennial, but it can be grown successfully as an annual in warmer parts of the temperate zones. Cuttings or smaller plants can be brought inside over the winter. They will usually go into a semi-dormant state and begin growing vigorously again when the weather warms up.

Cultivated varieties rarely produce viable seed, so they are propagated almost entirely by stem cuttings. Cuttings should be taken from hardened woody stems and be at least six inches

Chaya, Tree Spinach
Cnidoscolus aconitifolius,
C. chayamansa

long. They are easily rooted in damp soil. The stems should be dried for a few days and planted with the top of the cutting sticking about two-thirds of the way out of the soil. The stem cuttings can be started directly in the garden or field but usually do better when transplanted out after they have developed a root system. Keep young plants mulched to reduce competition from weeds. Once established, plants are very self-reliant and drought resistant. There is more danger from overwatering and waterlogging than from drought. Chaya is not much bothered by insect attacks; any damage is usually repaired quickly by new leaf growth.

With good conditions, chaya is impressively productive. Yields of 200 pounds of fresh leaf per 100-square-foot bed are possible, though half that is more likely. Frequent pruning makes for easier harvest and encourages the growth of side shoots, which increases leaf yield. Delay leaf harvest until chaya is at least 2 feet tall. After it is well established, you can harvest some leaves once a week. Chaya can be grown intensively, as a hedge, or as an attractive yard shrub.

Chaya is one of the most nutritious of all leafy vegetables, with high levels of protein, iron, calcium, vitamin A, and vitamin C. Compared to spinach, chaya contains nearly double the protein and vitamin A, four times the calcium, and seven times as much vitamin C. Some preliminary studies have suggested a possible role for chaya leaves in combating diabetes.[1]

Because raw chaya leaves contain a small amount of the toxin hydrocyanic acid, they should always be cooked for at least five minutes. This completely removes the toxin and provides a large margin of safety.

While people will understandably avoid foods that contain toxins, a bit of perspective here may be helpful. Many familiar foods have some degree

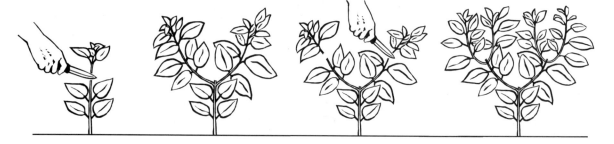

Cut off growing tip of plant to encourage new side shoots.

of hydrocyanic acid toxicity. These include almonds, millet, lima beans, and bamboo shoots. Most dried beans and grains need to be cooked to make them safe to eat.

Plants often use toxic compounds to discourage insects and larger animals from eating them. Clever humans learned ways to bypass many of the plants' defenses by cooking them. This hugely increased the range of quantity, quality, and variety of food available to us.

So the question is this: does a plant's value justify the effort needed to prepare it for eating? Chaya is an attractive, easy-to-grow perennial plant, little bothered by pests (for the reason explained above). Cooked chaya leaves are tasty and extremely nutritious. I think chaya is clearly worth the effort to prepare and can become a stellar addition to many home gardens.

Cranberry Hibiscus (Hibiscus acetosella)

Cranberry hibiscus is a short-lived perennial native to tropical Africa. It can be grown as an annual in most of the temperate zone. It is a beautiful plant with a range of deep magenta or burgundy-colored leaves and stems. The leaves have a bright tangy flavor and are a colorful and nutritious addition to salads or stir fries. The rich red color fades quickly when the leaves are boiled.

Cranberry hibiscus can be started from seeds or from stem cuttings. Seeds can be sown directly in garden beds after the soil warms in the spring, but will likely do better from transplanted seedlings. They can be started a few weeks before the last frost and set out when they are 5 inches tall. Spacing the plants three feet apart allows them room to grow. In warmer climates, a closer spacing can be used to create an attractive hedge. Pruning will encourage a more compact, bushier plant with more foliage.

In cooler climates, it needs to be replanted or overwintered inside. A few stem cuttings can be started in the fall and carried over inside to get a fast start when the soil warms up in the spring. Cuttings can be started in loose soil or in water. A few eight-inch stems put in a vase instead of flowers will quickly develop roots. The rooted cuttings

Cranberry Hibiscus,
Hibiscus acetosella

can be transplanted into the garden, but will usually rot if left in water for more than ten days.

Cranberry hibiscus may survive a frost but will be killed by hard freezing. In areas with mild winters, a heavy mulch may be enough to protect the roots and allow the plant to re-emerge in the spring. It rarely flowers or sets seed in climates with less than a 180-day growing season. It has a long taproot that benefits from deep soil and good drainage.

Garlic Chives, Chinese Chives (Allium tuberosum)

Garlic chives are a perennial member of the onion family. They are native to Asia, and are a popular vegetable in China, Japan, and Vietnam. They are easy to grow and the thin strap-like leaves can be harvested three or more times a year. In warm climates they can produce leaves year round. In colder climates they will die back completely to the ground over winter and the roots will re-sprout in the spring.

Garlic chives can be started from seed in early spring or by dividing a clump of roots at almost any time. Seed should not be over one year old. They are not fussy about soil. These plants can sometime spread vigorously, so some gardeners prefer to grow them in containers or where they can't easily escape to other parts of the garden. Surrounding them with grass is one strategy for containing their exuberant growth. Regular harvesting is another. Growing garlic chives interspersed with tomatoes reportedly reduces the problem of bacterial wilt in the tomatoes.

Garlic chives bloom with attractive, small star-shaped white flowers on tall stems in late summer. The flowers are excellent at attracting bees and butterflies. Given a reasonable amount of care, they can provide flavorful greens for soups, salads, and other dishes for ten years before needing to be replanted. They can be used as either a culinary herb or a green leafy vegetable and provide the same health benefits as garlic.

Garlic Chives,
Allium tuberosum

Jute, Molokhia (Corchorus olitorius)

Jute is a fast-growing annual plant that is probably native to Africa. It is grown both as a leaf vegetable and as a source of jute, or burlap, fiber. It is one of the leading leaf vegetables in much of Africa and is also widely grown and eaten in the Caribbean, Brazil, India, Bangladesh, China, Japan, and the Middle East. It can grow over six feet tall but is usually pruned to be kept at a convenient height for harvesting. Varieties of this plant grown for jute fiber are quite different from the leaf vegetable varieties and can grow up to 16 feet tall.

Jute prefers hot and humid conditions. It stops growing at temperatures below 60°F. Because it is a fast-growing plant, good harvests can be obtained in warmer temperate regions as well throughout most of the tropics. In Kentucky (where I garden), at 37° north latitude, it thrives especially well if started with some protection a couple of weeks earlier than other frost-sensitive plants. Until it is well established, jute benefits from a steady supply of soil moisture whether from rainfall or irrigation. It prefers sandy loam soils rich in organic matter and grows poorly on heavy clay.

Jute, Bush Okra,
Jute Mallow,
Jew's Mallow,
Molokhia, *Corchorus olitorius*

Seeds germinate better if immersed in nearly boiling water for five seconds before planting. Jute can be seeded directly in the home garden but usually does better if transplanted from seedlings. When seedlings are four inches tall, set them out in the garden bed about ten inches apart in rows about 20 inches apart. Jute is a good cut-and-come-again plant, with the first leaf harvest usually taken four to six weeks after transplanting. Keeping the plants pruned to a height of three to four feet above the ground stimulates the development of side shoots. Leaves can often be harvested every three weeks, up to eight times. Yields of 100 pounds per 100-square-foot bed are possible.

Jute is generally not bothered much by insect pests other than Japanese beetles, but is very susceptible to root-knot nematodes in warmer climates. Allowing adequate spacing for good air movement between plants reduces the likelihood of viral or fungal attack. Yields depend greatly on soil fertility, but repeated harvesting consistently out-produces harvesting the plants all at once.

Jute leaves are very perishable and need to be cooked and eaten, refrigerated, or dried shortly after harvest. They have a slightly bitter flavor and when cooked are mucilaginous (slimy) like okra. Thus, jute leaves (fresh or dried) are valued for their ability to thicken soups and stews. They are frequently available either frozen or dried in Asian and Middle Eastern grocery stores. Some variation on the word "molokhaya" is most often used on the label. In Africa, it is often prepared with black-eyed peas, pumpkin, or sweet potato with lime juice and chilis. Jute is one of the most nutritious vegetables, being especially rich in iron, calcium, folate, beta-carotene, and vitamin C.

Moringa, Horseradish Tree, Drumstick Tree, Malungay (Moringa oleifera, M. stenopetala)

Moringa is the name of a genus of 13 tropical and semi-tropical shrubs and trees that has attracted a great deal of interest over the past decade or so. Of the 13, *Moringa oleifera* is by far the most commonly grown for food. Originally from the foothills of the Himalayas, it has been cultivated in India for thousands of years. Over the past 50 years, it has quickly spread throughout the world's tropical zones.

Moringa stenopetala is originally from East Africa. It is less well known, and its area of cultivation has not spread nearly as wide or fast as *M. oleifera*. The African moringa has larger, somewhat milder-flavored leaves. It is more drought resistant but less cold hardy and also slower growing than its Indian cousin.

Moringa is valued because it is fast-growing, drought resistant, and has multiple uses. It leaves are eaten as a nutritious potherb; its seeds can be used to help purify water and yield a useful oil; its flowers are used to make tea; and its roots have been used as a substitute for horseradish. Moringa leaves are a potentially important source of many nutrients in the

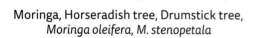

Moringa, Horseradish tree, Drumstick tree, *Moringa oleifera, M. stenopetala*

dryer, warmer parts of the world where malnutrition is rampant. The ability to produce an inexpensive local food during the dry season when little else is available has earned moringa such nicknames as "the tree of life" or "the miracle tree."

These accolades were not lost on health food marketers in wealthier countries. Imported moringa products, most often from India, are beginning to show up everywhere in North America and Europe. The enthusiasm for moringa is well-grounded, even if the prices for many moringa products are not. Moringa leaves are one of the most nutritious foods on the planet. The "miracles" of better health, however, are generally reserved for the malnourished women and children for whom moringa leaves can indeed be a life-saving food.

The tree is capable of extremely high yields and is very easy to grow—in the tropics. In climates cooler than zone 9, growing moringa is far more challenging. There are two basic approaches to growing moringa in temperate climates. Grow it as an annual during the hot summer, or grow it in a heated greenhouse, where it is protected from freezing temperatures and provided with adequate light over the winter. Growing moringa in a greenhouse is usually best done in a large container or a barrel cut in half. Moringa can be grown outdoors as an annual from zones 6 to 9.

Edible leaves are all that moringa offers gardeners in temperate climates. The relative warmth and long growing season of zone 9 is required to produce flowers, pods, and seeds. And using moringa roots as a substitute for horseradish is now widely discouraged because of toxins present in the bark of the root. That leaves leaves.

To produce a reasonable crop of moringa greens, plant seeds indoors in loose potting soil around the time of the last frost. When the soil warms up above 70°F, the baby moringas should be about six inches tall and ready to be transplanted into the garden. They will appreciate being planted in as warm and sunny a spot as you can find. They can be grown as a dense stand by setting out one seedling every 12 inches in rows 18 inches apart; then prune them back every three weeks or so. The highest yields of leaves have come from repeated cuttings of even denser plantings, but these require plenty of warm sunshine and more attention to fertilizing and irrigating.

Moringa can also be can be grown as individual trees and be allowed to spread out. With either approach, it important to keep moringa well pruned.

When grown for leaves, the leading tip of the plant (apical meristem) can be clipped off when the plant gets over three feet high, and side branches clipped off at two feet long. This encourages vigorous branching, maximum leaf production, and easy harvesting. Without any pruning, moringa will quickly make a tall, spindly tree (up to 30 feet high) with leaves only near the top.

Moringa is quite adaptable to different soil types. It is very drought resistant once established but won't tolerate waterlogging. Like most plants, moringa will produce far more foliage when grown in soil with adequate organic matter, nitrogen, and phosphorus. Moringa has relatively few problems with disease or pests, though it can be attacked by grasshoppers. Its leaves are tasty to most animals, and young plants may need protection from deer, rabbits, and groundhogs.

Moringa leaves are small and easily stripped off the stem. They can be eaten raw or cooked. Raw moringa has a little "bite," like mustard or radish. This is not surprising, as they contain similar beneficial antioxidant compounds. Like spinach, the mild flavor of lightly cooked moringa adapts to a wide variety of soups, stews, curries, omelets, and other dishes. It is important to pick the stems from the moringa leaves carefully, as any remaining stems make for wiry and unpleasant eating.

Moringa leaves have a lower moisture content than most other leafy vegetables. This makes them easy to preserve with solar dryers or electric food dehydrators. When dried below 10 percent moisture and kept cool and well sealed, it will remain in good condition for a full year. Finely ground dried moringa leaf is a potent source of convenient nutrition.

The extra effort that is required to grow tropical moringa in cooler climates is justified by the bounty of flavorful greens that can be produced through the heat of the summer. Because moringa leaf is so rich in protein, iron, calcium, magnesium, potassium, vitamins A and C, and especially in protective antioxidants, it could be one of the brightest stellar additions to your garden.

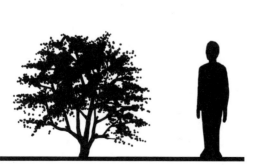

Unpruned and pruned moringa.

Moringa Plant Growth-Stimulant Spray

Freshly squeezed juice from the leaves of young moringa contains hormones that stimulate the growth of many types of plants. Studies in Nicaragua showed promising increases in yield and a shorter time to maturity in both corn and coffee trials.[2] The method described below was adapted from those studies.

1. Grind or pulp four cups of fresh young moringa shoots with a cup of water.
2. Put the pulped leaves in a strong cloth bag and squeeze out as much liquid as possible.
3. Dilute the moringa leaf juice with water. A cup of leaf juice should be diluted to make about two gallons of spray. Spray it onto the leaves of garden plants in the morning or evening.
4. Plants can be sprayed several times during the growing season, beginning about two weeks after germination.

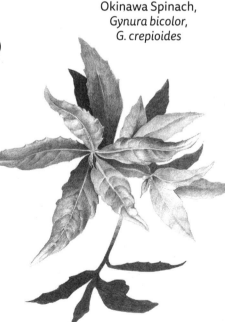

Okinawa Spinach,
Gynura bicolor,
G. crepioides

Okinawa Spinach, Gynura (Gynura bicolor, Gynura crepioides)

Okinawa spinach is a perennial plant in the huge aster family. It is native to the humid tropics of southeast Asia, and that is still the region where it is primarily grown and eaten. It will be killed back to the ground by a hard freeze but will often re-sprout in the spring when the soil warms, especially if given a protective mulch cover. Okinawa spinach produces edible leaves quickly enough to grow as an annual vegetable in temperate areas with a hot summer. Gynura is an excellent yard plant and is often grown as an edible ornamental due to its striking foliage that has glossy green upper sides and bright purple lower sides. It grows in clumps, quickly reaching three feet in diameter and three feet in height.

The leaves are nutritious and regrow rapidly, making it an exemplary cut-and-come-again home garden vegetable. Regular pruning stimulates further leaf production. It is almost always propagated by cuttings, which take a week or so to root and four or five weeks to reach harvest size. It prefers well-drained soil with plenty of added organic matter. Once established, Okinawa spinach grows fast enough and densely enough to hold its own against weeds. It is bothered little by pests or disease. It can produce 50 pounds of greens per year from a 100-square-foot bed if harvested weekly.

Once harvested, the quality of the leaves declines rapidly unless they are refrigerated. Okinawa spinach is sometime eaten raw in salads, but it is more often steamed, stir-fried, or added to soups and stews. It has a strong and distinctive but pleasant flavor often described as "piney." It is frequently mixed with milder greens to keep it from overwhelming the flavor of prepared dishes.

Taioba, Tannia, Malanga, Yautia (Xanthosoma sagittifolium); Belembe, Tannier Spinach (Xanthosoma brasiliense); Taro (Colocasia esculenta)

These are three members of the aroid, or elephant ear, family. Taioba and belembe are native to the Amazon region of South America, while taro originated in southeastern Asia. Tannia and taro are grown primarily for their starchy underground stems, or corms, that are eaten like potatoes. The leaves of tannia or malanga are often called "taioba," especially in southern Brazil, where they are an especially popular vegetable. Closely related belembe is grown only for its leaves.

Taioba, belembe, and taro are spectacular-looking plants, with their giant glossy green arrow-shaped leaves held high by slender curving stems. All three plants protect their leaves with sharp crystals of calcium oxalate and enzymes that irritate the mouth and throat of animals (including humans) that eat them. As leaf crops, belembe is considered the tastiest of the three, followed by taioba, and then taro leaves. The flavor preference reflects the declining levels of irritants in the three leaf crops. Both the crystals and the enzymes are usually rendered harmless by 10–15 minutes cooking. As you might imagine, they are rarely eaten raw.

All three plants are tropical perennials, and tannia and taro need at least ten months of warm weather to produce good crops of starchy corms. However, they can all be grown as annual leaf crops in the temperate zone. The

University of Massachusetts has a successful program introducing commercial production of taioba, a vegetable in great demand among the state's quarter-million Brazilian residents. The school is in USDA plant hardiness zone 5 at 42° north latitude. One difficulty for temperate-zone growers of these crops is locating good planting material. They are all usually propagated vegetatively from pieces of corm.

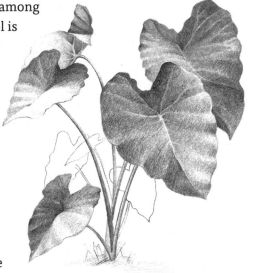

Taioba, Tannia,
Malanga, Yautia,
Xanthosoma sagittifolium

All three of these plants like wet soil, and some varieties of taro are purposely flooded. Taioba thrives in drier soil conditions and is more shade tolerant than taro. It is also less bothered by pests and diseases. Tannia and taro are often planted in mounds or ridges, but that is mainly to facilitate corm harvest and may not be helpful in growing the plants solely as leaf crops. Spacing the plants three feet apart allows adequate room to grow.

Young taioba leaves have better flavor than older ones. The center rib of the leaf is usually removed and the main lateral leaf veins are sometimes removed. Be careful not to get juice from raw aroid leaves in your eyes when handling taioba, as it is irritating. You can get a good idea how long you have to cook the leaves by tasting them. If they still have an irritating feeling in your mouth, they need to be cooked for a little longer.

Taioba and belembe are widely regarded as perhaps the most delicious of all greens. They are a good source of many essential nutrients including iron, calcium, vitamin A, vitamin C, and folate.

Tampala, Leaf Amaranth, Joseph's coat (Amaranthus tricolor)

Although the grain amaranths evolved in Central America and the foothills of the Andes Mountains in South America, the most familiar leaf amaranth species is native to south Asia. *Amaranthus tricolor* is an annual leaf crop that was domesticated in prehistoric times. It quickly grows up to three feet high. Varieties with bright red, yellow, and green leaves are grown throughout the world as ornamentals. Like maize and sugar cane, it uses the C4 photosynthetic pathway, which makes it especially efficient at producing food in bright sunlight and high temperatures. It is one of the fastest-growing and most productive of all our food plants.

Tampala grows best in well-drained soils rich in organic matter. It is frost sensitive and doesn't do well in cool or shady conditions. It requires a steady supply of water and may flower prematurely if the soil is allowed to dry out completely between rains. Soluble nitrogen fertilizers should be avoided because amaranth can become excessively high in nitrates.

Tampala usually germinates in three to five days and begins flowering in about five weeks. Seed is usually broadcast thinly over a bed or sown in narrow rows, 5–10 inches apart. Seedlings are prone to damping off and don't transplant well. The bed may need to be weeded once before the amaranth creates its own cover. It is subject to attack by a fairly wide range of insects, though nematodes and viruses are rarely a problem.

Where it is grown commercially, amaranth is usually uprooted or cut at ground level after three to four weeks. Pinching the lead stems will cause it to branch out and increase the number of partial leaf harvests, and thus the total yield. Yields can be up to 440 pounds of edible greens from a 100-square-foot garden bed.

Amaranthus tricolor is very nutritious as a cooked leaf vegetable. It is rich in protein, iron, calcium, magnesium, and vitamins A and C. Oxalic acid content can limit the availability of minerals. Nitrates can be kept lower if you don't use any synthetic nitrogen fertilizer; removing stems before cooking will also lower nitrates. In any case, unless more than one half pound per day is consumed, these anti-nutrients are unlikely to be a problem.

Toon, Chinese Mahogany, Fragrant Spring Tree, Red Toon, Chinese Cedar (*Toona sinensis*)

Toon is among the most unusual food crops in the world. Growing up to 65 feet tall, it is a tree whose principal food product is neither fruit nor nuts, but a leaf vegetable. Toon leaves were rated as the most nutritious of all vegetables and the highest in protective antioxidants by the World Vegetable Center in Taiwan. Grown both as a commercial food crop and as an ornamental yard tree, toon also produces fine quality wood that is prized for making sitars and electric guitars. That's a lot of street cred!

As some of its many names suggest, toon is originally from China and surrounding parts of Asia. It is the most cold hardy member of a plant family that includes mahogany and neem, a tree that produces highly valued organic insecticides and repellants. Toon can be grown as a long-living shade tree, as a hedge, or as a row crop. In northern China it is commonly grown in unheated plastic hoop houses or high tunnels to meet the growing demand for the vegetable.

Toon will grow in USDA zones 5–9, though it may struggle a bit in the coldest and warmest parts of those zones. It can be propagated by seed or from root suckers that sprout up near the base of established toon trees. Seeds should be less than a year old and usually need three months of winter chilling before they will germinate. Soak seeds overnight in warm water then plant in loose potting soil. They should sprout in about one week and can be set out as soon as the soil warms up.

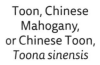

Toon prefers deep, well-drained soil (who doesn't?); it grows better in fertile sandy soils than in heavy clay soils. It is not particular about pH or rainfall. Saplings need protection from freezes and drought, but, once established, they need very little care. If you are primarily interested in the edible leaves, keep toon pruned back to a height of 6–8 feet. This makes for easy harvest

Toon, Chinese Mahogany, or Chinese Toon, *Toona sinensis*

and promotes vigorous leaf production on lateral shoots. Root suckers (saplings) will likely sprout up near the base of the original tree within two years. New toon trees can be started by carefully severing the root suckers from the parent tree with a sharp spade. They can then be dug up with a bit of soil and transplanted elsewhere. Alternatively, root suckers can be left alone and will often form a dense and productive clump.

There are two basic varieties of the plant, green toon and red toon. The red varieties have dramatic foliage in the spring, with colors ranging from deep reds and purples to psychedelic pinks. The green varieties, in contrast, have bronze-colored spring leaves. The leaves of both types turn a glossy green in summer and to yellows and golds in autumn before falling with the onset of cold weather. After its first year, toon usually forms flowers by July. They are very sweet scented and hang in white or pink clusters.

The Chinese happily eat both, but the purple or red leaves are widely considered to be milder and have better texture. Two varieties, 'Flamingo' and 'Red North,' are thought to be especially tasty. (Not everyone would use the word "tasty" to describe toon leaves. They have a pronounced flavor reminiscent of roasted garlic or onions.) Toon is rarely eaten raw, but it adds a pleasant flavor to soups and eggs. Toon is a traditional ingredient in many Chinese New Year's dishes. Toon leaves are sometimes dried or salted for export, and a toon leaf tea that tastes like thin onion soup is thought to promote good health.

Harvest leaves when they are young and tender. As the leaves mature, they become more fibrous and the flavor intensifies out of the edibility range. Toon leaves are decidedly an acquired taste, but they are a taste worth acquiring. Produced in abundance on beautiful trees, toon leaves are perhaps the most nutritious of all vegetables and a star waiting to take root in your garden. Plus, you can make your next guitar from the wood if you don't acquire the taste.

Vine Spinach (*Basella alba, B. rubra*)

Vine spinach is a perennial plant with mild-flavored, somewhat mucilaginous leaves. *Basella alba* refers to green stemmed varieties, and *Basella rubra* to varieties with reddish stems and leaves, but they are essentially the same species of plant. Basella is native to south Asia, the word apparently comes from the Singhalese language of Sri Lanka.

Vine spinach is a heat-loving tropical that grows slowly—if at all—in cool weather and is easily killed by frost. It shouldn't be planted outdoors until night temperatures are consistently warm. Vine spinach can be grown in the warmer temperate zones, especially if it is given a head start of a few weeks in a greenhouse or cold frame. It tends to start slowly but then grows very quickly once the weather becomes too warm for other greens. It will survive in most soils but does best in rich soil with high organic matter content.

Vine spinach can be planted very close together. If you use a one-inch spacing, you will need to thin it out to allow one or two strong plants every foot or so, and the thinnings make good salad greens. Vine spinach can be propagated by stem cuttings as well as seed, and will often spontaneously form new roots where the plant touches soil. A few pieces of stem at least 6 inches long may be started in potting soil so that some

Vine Spinach,
Malabar Spinach,
*Basella alba,
B. rubra*

plants are ready to transplant into the garden when it starts getting too hot for cool-weather crops.

Vine spinach is an attractive plant most often grown on trellises or fences. It can be grown without a trellis, but it has a strong vining habit and forms a somewhat tangled mess if allowed to run freely on the ground. Leaves grown on trellises are much less likely to be contaminated by soil bacteria from splashing rain. This is especially important when the leaves are eaten raw in salads. A variation is to grow vine spinach in hanging baskets and harvest the stems before they reach the ground. It is especially important that vine spinach growing in containers be watered regularly.

After three or four weeks of growth, vine spinach will benefit from harvesting of leaves and stem as often as every ten days, as this stimulates the growth of new shoots. Vine spinach is surprisingly free of insect pests for a plant with such tender leaves and stems, though it is prone to nematode damage in warmer climates.

In Kentucky, which has a six-month growing season, the smaller-leafed *B. rubra* reliably produces viable seed and plentiful volunteers the following spring, but the larger-leafed *B. alba* is usually killed by frost before its seeds are mature. The red-stemmed *B. rubra* produces edible leaf in early and mid-summer, while the green stemmed *B. alba* does most of its leaf production in late summer and early fall.

Yields of vine spinach vary a great deal depending on the climate, soil, and cultivation techniques employed. High yields are possible, and yields of over 300 pounds of greens from a 100-square-foot bed have been recorded in a six-month growing season. Vine spinach is mild flavored, and even after flowering begins, the young leaves are tender and mild enough to eat raw in salads. It is often cooked with garlic, ginger, curry, and other strong-flavored herbs and spices. Vine spinach leaves are useful for thickening soups. Their intensely purple fruits are sometimes used to color rice for special occasions.

Vine spinach is a very nutritious vegetable. On a dry-weight basis, it is in the same elevated category as moringa or chaya. Moringa leaves are about 79 percent moisture, while vine spinach leaves are 93% moisture. This means that 100 grams (3.5 ounces) of fresh moringa will have 21 grams of dry matter, and 100 grams of vine spinach will have only 7 grams. When both are fully dried, though, vine spinach leaves will have a very similar nutritional profile to moringa leaves, with somewhat less protein and iron but more calcium, vitamin A, vitamin C, and folate. However, because they are mucilaginous, vine spinach leaves are more difficult to dry than leaves with low moisture content, such as moringa leaves.

Vine spinach is extremely low in calories while being rich in nutrients, including protein. To illustrate, 100 calories of beefsteak provides 6 grams of protein, while 100 calories of vine spinach will supply 14 grams of protein. This makes it a great food for losing weight while still getting the protein you need. Still, the real beauty of vine spinach is that it provides abundant, mild-tasting greens through the heat of the summer, when few others are available.

Walking Stick Kale (*Brassica oleracea* var. *longata*)

In the diffuse light of the long cool summer days of the British Isles, a cabbage of heroic proportions evolved. It had various names. It was called walking stick kale for the strong, lightweight walking sticks that were made from its stalk; Jersey cabbage for the Jersey Islands where it prospered; or tree collards, because it could grow up to 18 feet tall. It is a perennial member of the cabbage family that can be started from seeds or from cuttings. It typically takes two years to reach a height of 6–10 feet, though it can sometimes grow up to 10 feet tall in just six months. Walking stick kale has been known to provide greens for up to 20 years—if it is well cared for and doesn't encounter extreme hot or cold weather.

Unless it is being grown as a novelty, it is usually pruned to encourage branching at a height that can be reasonably reached without a ladder. At the top of the stem, a cap of large grayish-green collard-like leaves develop. These can be plucked regularly and will regrow. Leaves are best picked from oldest to newest when they are about 6 inches long, starting with the lower ones and moving up. This encourages the plant to grow taller. Side shoots will form where the leaf stems have been cut.

Walking Stick Kale,
Jersey Kale,
Brassica oleracea
var. *longata*

Seed is often started indoors about five weeks before the average last frost so that good growth can be made before hot summer temperatures set in. This plant prefers fertile soil with plenty of nitrogen and a pH that is neutral or even slightly alkaline. It suffers from most of the usual cabbage family pests (cabbage worms, flea beetles, club root) and responds to most of the organic gardening treatments for them. A strong support pole at least 6 feet tall will help to prevent the plant from falling or blowing over.

These giant members of the cabbage family were known as excellent feed for cattle and other livestock, but were also a food of the peasantry. The stalks, left to air dry for ten months, were used as a substitute for scarce wood in many applications. However, the greatest value of the plants was as a source of protective antioxidants, protein, calcium, iron, and vitamins A, C, and K in the diets of the people of the Jersey Islands. Its high vitamin C content was especially important in preventing scurvy, a relatively common problem in such northern latitudes. Walking stick kale provides an abundant and reliable source of highly nutritious and tasty greens that can be harvested year round. It is heartening to see recent renewed interest in this giant perennial leaf crop, after a long stretch of neglect and diminished social status.

Invasive Plants

There is always some risk of inadvertently introducing an invasive species when we add a new crop to the garden, and it is important to minimize that risk. "Invasive species" is a wildly imprecise term, but it generally refers to a species that is outside its natural distribution area and threatens biological diversity.

It is more than a bit ironic to be warning against invasive introductions as a member of a species that originated in East Africa and now is colonizing Antarctica and leaving garbage on the moon. Still, managing invasive plant species is a passionately controversial subject for botanists, conservationists, and agriculturalists. Most would agree that gardeners have a responsibility to check local lists of prohibited and potentially invasive plant species before introducing plants, as well as an obligation to closely watch any new plants for signs of uncontrollable reproduction.

Plants compete for habitat, sunlight, water, and soil minerals like companies compete for market share. A plant species with a significant survival advantage can quickly become invasive in much the same way that supercenters displace Mom and Pop stores, or digital cameras displace film cameras. We may miss the variety and character of the little stores, and the vitality of the community may suffer, but it is hard to control the Invisible Hand. People travel far, fast, and frequently, and often inadvertently bring scraps of alien genetic code into new environments. Most of the time, the results are harmless. Sometimes they are positive, as with a new flower or delicious food crop; and sometimes they are damaging botanical invasions. It is prudent to take precautions and try to prevent the invasions, but it is also reasonable to accept that life is opportunistic and not easily corralled.

Without dismissing the very real danger from invasive plants, it seems worth noting that biodiversity is a two-way street. Our food-growing lands have been systematically stripped of diversity, and that lack of diversity has been enforced by heavy use of bio-cides. Reversing that trend will require the careful introduction of new species of food plants, not just slightly different varieties or cultivars of the small handful of species that we now grow. Adventurous gardeners can take part in this effort by creating millions of small pockets of increased biodiversity.

For starters, gardeners can begin to infuse the roughly 40 millions of acres of simple lawnscapes in the US with food-producing polycultures. As they repair depleted soil and establish more complex plantings on their small parcels, gardeners can make room within the human habitat for other creatures. More diverse communities of birds, amphibians, reptiles, worms, bacteria, fungi, and other living beings will quickly reinhabit the neighborhood. One can only hope that this more biologically friendly approach will eventually be extended to the millions of acres of herbicide-scoured corn and soybeans. Talk about invasive!

PART III

Some More
Advanced Techniques

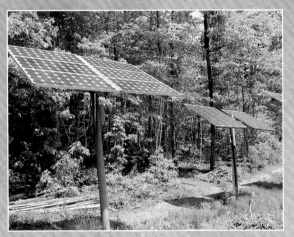

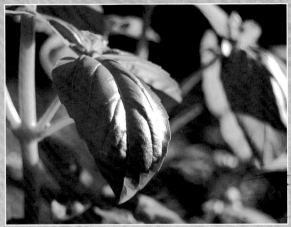

Above: Mechanical and biological solar energy collectors

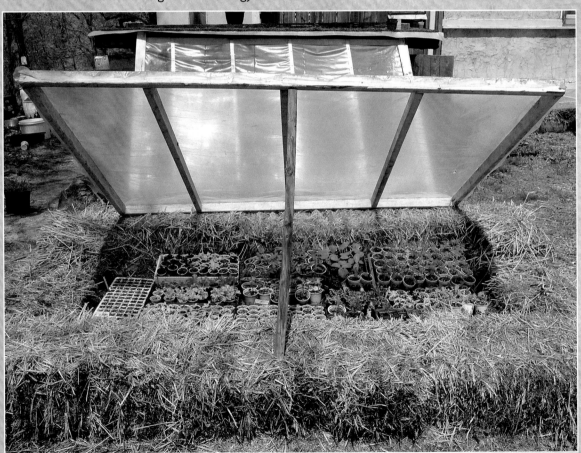

Starting sets in a straw bale insulated hotbed

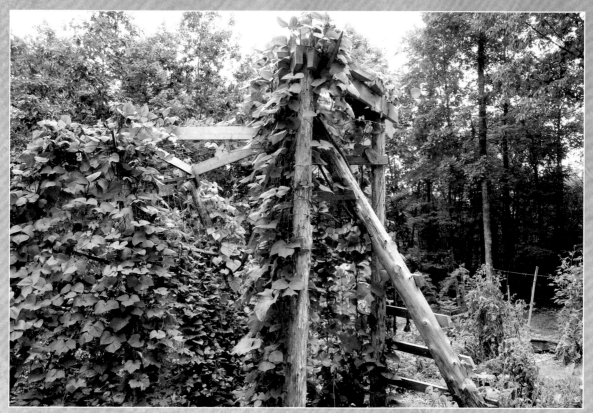

Above: Vine spinach, gourds, hyacinth beans, and rice beans climbing a large trellis

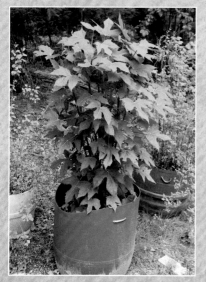

Chaya thriving in half a barrel

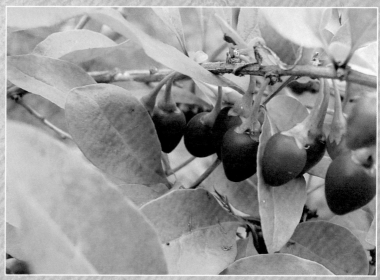

Goji berries with super-nutritious leaves

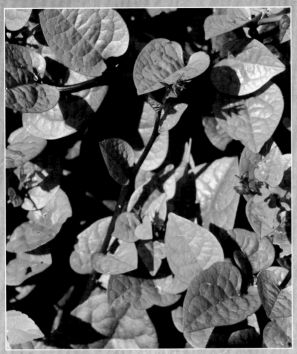

Above: Vine spinach (*Basella rubra*)

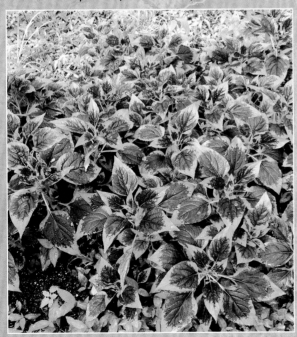

Quail grass (*Celosia argentea*)

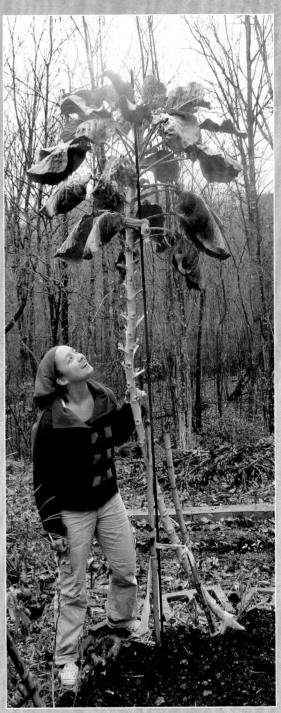

Walking stick kale (*Brassica oleracea longata*)

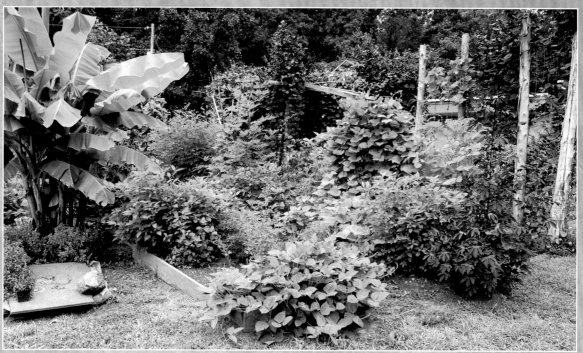
Above: Dense polyculture of leaf crops

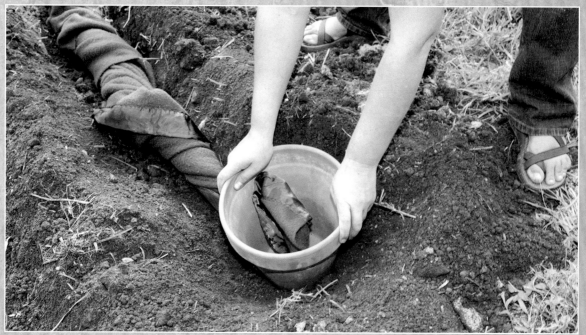
Installing wick irrigation in a garden bed

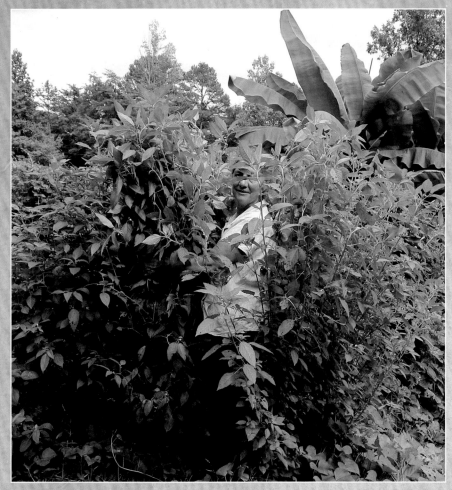

Left:
Bumper crop of
edible leaf jute
(*Corchorus olitorius*)

Below left:
Sweet potato slips
ready to transplant

Below right:
Nutritious leaves and
seeds from beautiful
Hopi amaranth
(*Amaranthus cruentus*)

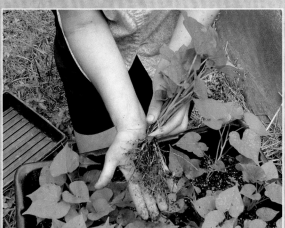

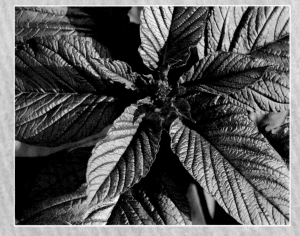

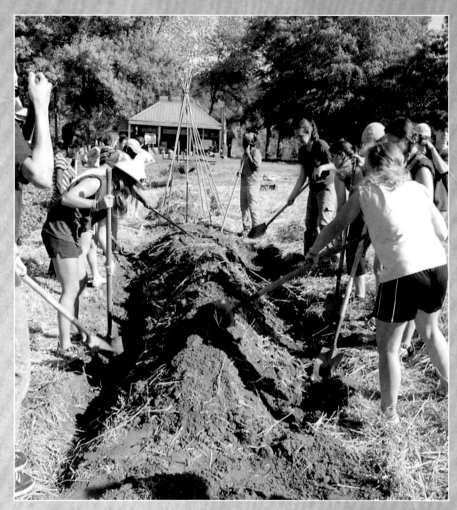

Top:
Building a raised
garden bed is fast
with many hands.

Lower left:
Vine spinach
snack bars

Lower right:
Making leaf
enriched pasta

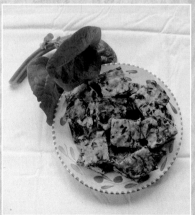

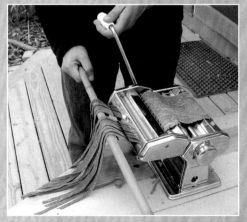

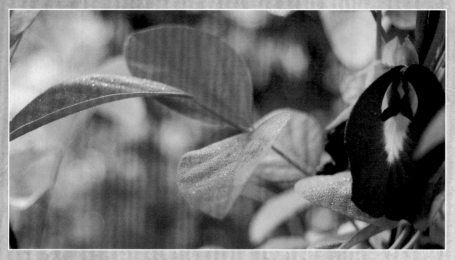

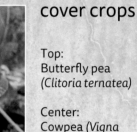

Edible leaf cover crops

Top:
Butterfly pea
(*Clitoria ternatea*)

Center:
Cowpea (*Vigna unguiculata*)

Lower left:
Winter peas and barley

Lower right:
Hyacinth bean
(*Lablab purpureus*)

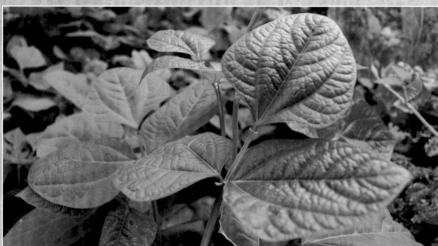

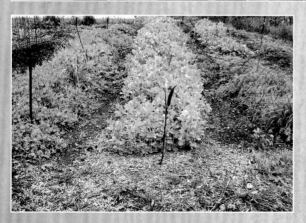

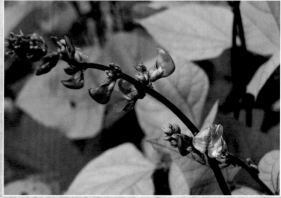

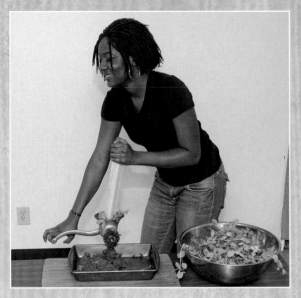

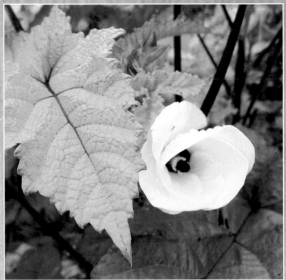

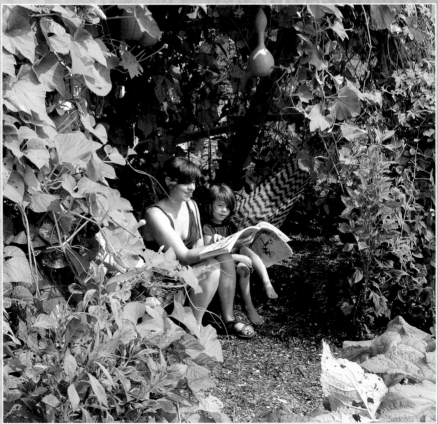

Above left:
Grinding leaves for
leaf concentrate

Above right:
West African okra
(*Abelmoschus caillei*)

Right:
Relaxing in the
shade of a leafy
home garden

8

Vegetable Versatility

❊ ❊ ❊

Growing Multi-Purpose Leaf Crops

The ability to obtain each of the nutrients we need from a wide variety of food sources has been an enormous evolutionary advantage for omnivorous humans. As hunters and gatherers, we may have had favorite game animals and favorite herbs and berries, but we normally ate a wide variety of foods to assure that we got the nutrients essential to our health. We carried this risk-averse approach into our days of subsistence farming, planting a variety of crops to avoid the disastrous consequences of a main crop failing. The economic value of spreading risk is the basis of all social insurance programs. Enlarging the biodiversity of our agricultural systems confers the same benefit of distributing the risk across many food crops.

In the specialized monocrop farming that currently produces almost all our food, the output of particular commodities is prodigious, while the labor costs are extremely low. Food-growing systems that integrate more species of plants and animals into production inevitably have greater labor and management costs. However, these more ecologically complex systems typically have higher total food output and far better protection against catastrophic crop failures.

The same diversity principle can be applied to individual plants. Most plants that we grow for food have more than one potential use. While commercial agriculture normally focuses on the single most profitable output from a plant, a sustainable system can make use of the whole plant. For example, we can eat both the sweet potato *and* its leaves. Having two nutritious

119

products from a single plant offers the grower an important advantage in food security. (This fact has not been lost on NASA, which is investigating both quinoa and cowpeas, two seed crops with edible leaves, as possible crops in their Controlled Ecological Life Support System for manned space flights of long duration.)

Not all plant leaves are edible, but a great many are. Virtually all crops are initially leaf crops, and finding additional uses for many food plants is often simply a matter of finding a way to make better use of their edible leaves. The point is to see the plants in their entirety, not as just a source of one particular product. This perspective offers the creative gardener a much wider range of botanical options for supper. Techniques, such as solar drying and making leaf concentrate that enable us to more effectively capture, preserve, and absorb the nutrients in green leaves, greatly improve the prospects for these multiple-use food plants.

There is clearly enormous potential in utilizing multiple parts of food plants. However, the structure of industrialized economies is such that labor-intensive techniques, like growing multi-use crops, have not been well researched. When they are considered at all, it is usually in the realm of subsistence farmers in tropical countries struggling with extreme poverty. This, unfortunately, is a group that gets very little good research done on its behalf. Cutting-edge North American horticulturists are in a position to develop some improved techniques that could have great benefit to these subsistence farmers, while at the same time shifting the shape of their own food experience. This is an area where informal networks of small farmers and home gardeners can take the lead. This sort of research doesn't require expensive lab equipment and research grants. Rather, it needs the sort of persistence and keen observation that good gardeners have in abundance. I would love to see open-source communities of kitchen gardeners make the results of their trials and errors available online. Ideally, regional growers associations and university departments would begin developing more rigorous databases keeping track of which varieties of which plants are best suited to partial leaf harvests, when to begin harvesting, and how much to harvest without undue loss of yield to the principal food being grown. It would be a true gift to the coming generations of growers.

In the meanwhile, I offer these basic guidelines as a starting point for growing multi-use leaf crops:

- Harvest no more than one-third of the leaves at one time so the plant can still produce an acceptable yield of the main crop. Almost all plants have some built-in margin of extra leaf production to compensate for animals browsing. Reduction of yield in the fruit or root typically begins when about 20 percent of the leaf is harvested.
  - Don't harvest leaves until the plant is at least three weeks old.
  - Harvest leaves before the plants flower.
  - Harvest leaves with a sharp knife or scissors to reduce risk of plant disease.
  - Leaves that are shaded by other leaves higher on the plant can usually be harvested without reducing yield of the main crop. This is also true for leaves that are shaded by other plants in the garden.
  - Record how much leaf you harvest, and when you harvest, to see how it affects yield of fruits, seed, and roots. The botany of each type of plant is different.

This section describes how to grow some of the plants that have edible leaves in addition to other uses and why they might be worth growing. The first and probably most important category of multi-use leaf crops—edible cover crops—is discussed in Chapter 11. Other important categories of multi-use leaf crops include staple food crops with edible leaves, traditional garden vegetables with edible leaves, and ornamental plants with edible leaves.

Staple Food Crops with Edible Leaves

Amaranth (Amaranthus hypochondriacus, A. cruentus and A. caudatus)

The name amaranth derives from a Greek word meaning "life everlasting." This may seem like an odd name for a plant family made up of mainly fast-growing annuals. Perhaps it referred to the plant's ability to readily reproduce itself from its abundant seed. Most of the world's roughly 500 species of amaranths are considered to be weeds; some are used as leafy vegetables or as ornamentals. One species grown exclusively for greens, tampala, *Amaranthus tricolor*, is discussed in Chapter 7.

In the Western Hemisphere, however, three types of amaranth seed became important staple foods. Two of the three amaranth species that have been grown for their grain, *A. hypochondriacus* and *A. cruentus*, are native to southern Mexico, while *A. caudatus* is native to the Andes region of South

America. Like quinoa and buckwheat, amaranth seed is sometimes called a pseudo-grain because it is the seed of a broadleaf plant that is eaten like a grain.

The grain amaranths were among the very first plants that were systematically improved by breeding. Aztec children sorted through piles of seed and separated out the occasional white seeds. These were grown in separate plots until varieties with only white seeds were developed. The white seeded amaranth had lower levels of tannin, and thus was milder tasting and more easily digested.

Production of grain amaranth declined even more sharply than quinoa after the Spanish conquest. It was estimated that 20,000 tons of grain amaranth were brought annually in tribute to Moctezuma, the Aztec Emperor in Tenochtitlan in the years preceding the conquest by Cortez. The Catholic Spanish banned the cultivation of amaranth because the ground amaranth seeds were sometimes mixed with human blood and shaped into snakes, birds, mountains, deer, or gods and eaten during Aztec religious ceremonies.

Grain amaranth is now making a modest resurgence in Latin America and northern India. It has also become a specialty health food product in North America and Europe. The amaranth pseudo-grain is far richer in protein than the true grains, and the protein has a surplus of the essential amino acid lysine which is deficient in corn, wheat, and rice.

All of the amaranths employ C4 photosynthetic metabolism. This is a variation on the photosynthetic system used by corn, sugar cane, sorghum, and other plants to maximize growth in hot, dry climates with intense sunlight. Broadleaf C4 plants are rare, and this attribute gives amaranth unusual drought tolerance for a shallow-rooted plant. Amaranths will grow in a wide range of soils but prefer sandy soils with good drainage and a slightly acidic pH. Most amaranths are sensitive to cold weather, but, among the grain am-

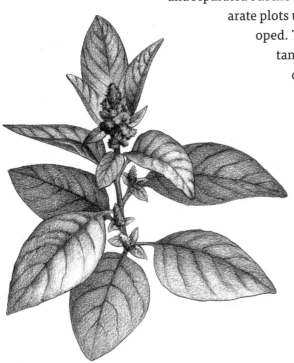

Amaranth,
Amaranthus cruentus,
A. hybridus,
A. hypochondriacus

aranths, *A. caudatus*, which developed high in the Andes Mountains, has some tolerance to cold.

The leaves of all the grain amaranths are sometimes eaten for greens. Sometimes the seed is over-planted and the thinnings are eaten as greens. *A. cruentus* has traditionally been grown as a combination leaf and seed crop. The Hopis in the US southwest developed brilliant red varieties of *A. cruentus* that produced well in that hot dry climate. It can be planted densely and thinned for greens, but also does well when the growing tips of the young plants are pinched off. This causes more lateral shoots to form, and these too can be pruned for greens. Leaves can be harvested at any time until seeds begin forming; unless the partial leaf harvest is too severe, the plants recover to produce bountiful heads of edible seed.

Enough leaves for a meal can be harvested from a small patch of *A. cruentus* every two to three weeks. This delays seed formation. Amaranth is a crop with tremendous potential for gardeners because it grows so quickly that it can often be planted after early garden crops are harvested or before fall crops are sown. It is easy to save *A. cruentus* seeds, and the plant often self-seeds the area where it has been grown. The volunteer seedlings can be easily transplanted into a more desirable spacing. This eliminates the cost of seeds.

Amaranth leaves are good sources of protein, calcium, iron, vitamin A, vitamin C, and folate. Although the seeds have more protein than any of the staple grains, on a dry-weight basis, the leaves are richer still, with three times as much protein as the seeds. Unfortunately, high levels of oxalic acid somewhat diminish the absorption of calcium. Don't use synthetic nitrogen fertilizers with amaranth because it results in excessively high amounts of nitrates in the leaves. Boiling amaranth leaves, then rinsing them will remove some of the nitrates.

Bean (Phaseolus vulgaris)

The common bean was domesticated in southern Mexico and in the Andes Mountains of South America over 6,000 years ago. It has at least 1,000 names and 10,000 varieties, including kidney bean, pinto bean, navy bean, cranberry bean, wax bean, green bean, black bean, and turtle bean. It has become a popular food throughout the world and is sometimes referred to as "The Poor Man's Meat" because of its high protein content.

Bean cultivars are either climbing pole types or dwarf bush type. The pole beans grow up to ten feet and require some sort of support or trellis. The bush varieties are less than three feet high and produce flowers and seeds much earlier in the season. Pole beans generally yield about twice as many beans as bush beans, but they take nearly twice as long to do so. Bush beans usually have lower labor costs and are often harvested all at one time for processing. Despite higher labor requirements, pole beans are often preferred for family gardens because they will produce a steady supply of beans over a much longer time.

The soil should be at least 54°F before planting beans; the ideal growing temperature is between 72–78°F. The common bean is sensitive to frost, waterlogging, soil acidity, salinity, and aluminum toxicity. Seeds are usually planted every two inches in rows 24–32 inches apart. Pole beans are often planted in groups of three or four at the base of whatever support they will be climbing. Before planting, seeds should be treated with a bacterial inoculant designated for beans (discussed in Chapter 11). There are several general purpose garden inoculants that will treat bean seed as well as many other legumes.

Beans are rarely grown solely as a cover crop because other plants that are less susceptible to insect and disease problems can fix more nitrogen. However, they are still frequently used as an *intercrop* with corn, sorghum, millet, and cassava, significantly reducing the fertilizer demand of those crops.

Outside of Africa and Indonesia, few people realize that beans also produce highly nutritious and tasty leaves for potherbs. Bean leaves are grown in two different ways. When grown as a separate crop for leaves, they are planted more densely than when grown for beans, and the plants are usually uprooted at three to five weeks. Like cowpeas, the plants can also be cut when about 8 inches tall, and allowed to regrow for a second cutting, though beans in general don't make strong regrowth.

Some varieties of beans have leaves that are too fibrous to make a good leaf crop, especially if grown in hot and dry conditions. Sometimes, farmers and gardeners try to combine a harvest of leaves and beans. This is best done by harvesting leaves from the lower third of the plant just before flowering begins. Bean leaves are very rich in beta-carotene, vitamin C, iron, calcium, and protein.

Quinoa (Chenopodium quinoa)

Quinoa (KEEN-wah) is native to the foothills of the Andes Mountains, where it has been grown for over 6,000 years. Considered a sacred plant by the Incas, quinoa production diminished greatly after the Spanish invasion. For the last 400 years, it has been a relatively minor regional crop. Recently, quinoa seed has gained popularity in the international health food market as an expensive alternative to rice and other true grains (seeds of annual grasses). It contains more total protein (12–18 percent) and a better balance of essential amino acids than true grains, which are all deficient in lysine. Quinoa also lacks gluten, a protein in wheat to which many people have an adverse reaction. A further advantage of quinoa over grains is that the starch granules in quinoa seed are very small and easily digested.

Along with spinach, beets, and Swiss chard, quinoa is a member of the Chenopodium family. While the seed is by far the more familiar food, quinoa greens have also been eaten and appreciated wherever the crop is grown. Young quinoa leaves are nearly indistinguishable from the greens of the common weed lambsquarters, and they make a potherb similar to spinach.

Quinoa is a hardy crop, growing at elevations up to 13,000 feet. It is tolerant of drought and saline soil, but produces much better with an even supply of moisture and deep, well-drained soil. The seeds sprout very quickly and are protected from birds and other animals by a coating of bitter saponins. When the seeds will be used for eating, these saponins are removed by rinsing or scrubbing the seeds before they are cooked.

Like the seeds, the quinoa greens are rich in protein. They also have higher levels of iron, calcium, vitamin A, and vitamin C. Unfortunately, like all the members of this family, quinoa has relatively high levels of oxalic acid in its leaves, which makes its calcium less readily absorbed in the human body. However, unless someone is genetically inclined to form kidney stones, a moderate amount of dietary oxalic acid in an otherwise adequate diet appears to be harmless.

Leaves for greens should be harvested before the plant flowers. Andean farmers thin overcrowded young plants and use the thinnings for greens. Careful partial harvest of leaves before seeds form will result in the highest total nutrient production for a given area. Optimizing systems for combined yield of quinoa leaf and seed harvest will likely depend on availability of labor and markets for the greens. Quinoa greens are usually eaten by the farmers as a fringe benefit or sold in local markets.

Sweet Potato (Ipomoea batatas)

Sweet potatoes are sprawling perennial plants that probably originated in Central America, where they have been cultivated for over 5,000 years. The crop is now grown throughout the tropics and the warmer parts of the temperate zone, where it is often grown as a long-season annual. Sweet potatoes are among the ten most important food crops in the world. However, because much of the crop is grown by subsistence farmers for home use rather than for commerce, research on sweet potatoes has been minimal.

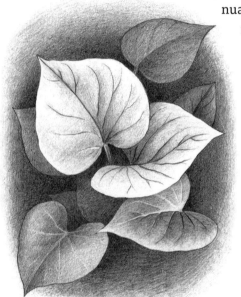

Sweet Potato,
Ipomoea batatas

It is an excellent dual-purpose food crop because its leaves are nutritious and widely eaten. Both tuber and leaves are rich in pro-vitamin A, folate, and calcium. The leaves are perhaps the best source of the antioxidant lutein, which is important in protecting our skin from sun damage and our eyes from age-related loss of vision.

In a system where both the leaves and tubers are well managed for high yield, sweet potatoes can probably produce more nutrients per acre than any other crop. They have one of the highest returns of nutrients—relative to the time and effort expended—of any crop.

Sweet potato grows best in loose sandy soil, but will thrive in any well-drained soil. It is a very frost-sensitive plant that requires at least 100 warm days to produce tubers of reasonable size. In cooler climates, black plastic is sometimes used to warm the soil, and floating row covers can help warm the air around the plants. However, even where the growing season is too short to get good yields of tubers, sweet potatoes can be grown for their leaves. High levels of nitrogen will favor foliage growth at the expense of tuber size. A slightly acid soil pH is ideal.

In the temperate zone, sweet potato plants are usually started from shoots that sprout from the sweet potato. Often called slips, these shoots are grown by placing whole or half sweet potatoes in a few inches of damp sand or by suspending the sweet potato in water. They should be started about six weeks before the last expected frost. They need to be kept warm during this time.

When shoots are 6–9 inches high, they can be gently twisted and pulled from the mother sweet potato and planted in the garden. Slips are usually planted 12–18 inches apart. Closer spacing results in more sweet potatoes, but smaller size, while wider spacing produces a smaller number of larger tubers. Sweet potatoes can also be grown closely spaced to smother weeds. When planted 6 inches apart or closer, they will quickly form a dense groundcover that is both attractive and edible. Though the yield of edible tubers will be small, this is a realistic way of removing tough perennial grasses or nutsedge from a garden or field without resorting to herbicides. Sweet potatoes are also one of the best edible greens to grow in containers or hanging baskets.

Once they are well established, up to one-third of the leaves can be harvested every three weeks. Earlier light or less frequent leaf harvests will result in greater tuber yield, but the maximum total food value will always come from combination of leaf and tuber harvesting. The stems of sweet potato are often eaten along with the leaves, but they offer little beyond water and fiber. Given good conditions for growth, up to 115 pounds of fresh sweet potato greens could be harvested from a 100-square-foot bed.

Sweet potato leaves are mild flavored and tender. In addition to making them good for supper, this makes them very delicious to deer and groundhogs, so they need some protection. Repeated spraying of the young leaves with diluted chili pepper sauce will discourage feeding. Although it is already one of the world's leading food crops, sweet potatoes have enormous potential that remains to be tapped. Flexible systems that optimize combined leaf and tuber yield need to be developed to realize that potential. Their ability to produce good yields with minimal fertilizer will become more crucial as energy prices inevitably escalate.

Traditional Garden Vegetables That Have Edible Leaves

Understandably, most North American gardeners are unaware of many of the interesting species of leaf crops grown in Asia and Africa. What is somewhat surprising is how few gardeners are aware that many of their traditional garden vegetable plants also have leaves that are tasty and nutritious. Beans, beetroot, okra, peas, peppers, pumpkins, onions, and turnips, all lend themselves to a partial harvest of their tasty nutritious leaves. There are no fixed rules for determining how the partial harvest of leaves impacts the yield of these traditional garden vegetables. Mastering the integration of multi-use crops into the garden is an engaging mix of botanical science, agricultural craft, and even a touch of artistry. Multi-use crops reward the observant and patient gardener. Some of the best multi-use garden plants are listed below.

The precautionary principle suggests that any new food added to the diet be eaten in small amounts to allow time to observe any possible allergenic or other adverse effects. This is especially true for young children. Using younger leaves and cooking them provides an additional margin of safety.

Beets (Beta vulgaris)

Beets are one of about 150 species of the Chenopodium family. Originally from the edges of the Mediterranean Sea, their coastal origin probably explains their high tolerance to salt in the soil. Grown for its leaves by ancient Romans, the use of the swollen beetroot came much later. Swiss chard and sugar beets are two familiar variations within the same beet species.

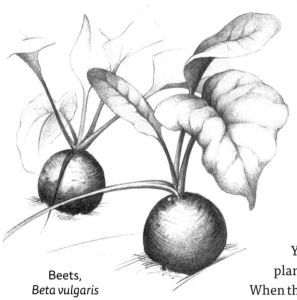

Beets have deep taproots that offer some protection from drought. What you find when you open a package of "beet seeds" are actually hard, dried fruits containing up to eight seeds. This accounts for the difficulty of getting uniform stands of beet seedlings. Beets can tolerate light frosts but grow best at temperatures between 60–70°F. They are somewhat more tolerant of hot weather than their close relative, spinach.

Loose sandy soil is preferred for roots, but heavier soil is fine for growing beet greens. Yield is reduced in acid soils. Beets can be planted every 2 inches in rows 10–16 inches apart. When they are 2–3 inches tall or when they begin to look

Beets,
Beta vulgaris

overcrowded, they may be thinned, and the thinnings eaten in salads or stir fries. Beets are a good container plant as long as the soil is at least 12 inches deep. They can be replanted every three to four weeks during the growing season to maintain a steady supply of small, tender beetroots and greens.

The strong red color present in most beets and some beet greens comes from betacyanin. This pigment is thought to have cancer-fighting properties, especially against colon cancer. Beet juice is sometimes used as a natural food coloring. Though beets are a very healthy food, they can cause alarmingly red urine (which is totally harmless).

Beet greens can be grown as a separate crop or as a by-product of growing the roots. Beetroot yields are usually acceptable even when up to one-third of the leaves are carefully harvested for greens. Cold weather and nitrogen-rich soil favor production of leaves at the expense of the edible roots. Compared with their roots, beet greens contain more than triple the iron, seven times the calcium, six times the vitamin C, and 150 times the vitamin A activity. Beet greens have a slightly coarser flavor and texture than spinach, but they can be prepared and enjoyed in most of the same ways.

Garlic (Allium sativum)

Garlic originated in Central Asia and has been cultivated in Egypt for over 4,000 years. It is now grown throughout most of the world. Garlic is a close relative of onion, and it also has a distinctive pungent flavor and aroma. The people of China and Korea produce over 70 percent of the world's garlic and eat enough garlic to consider it a vegetable, rather than a flavoring agent.

While primarily used as a flavoring for a great many dishes, garlic also has a rich history of use as a botanical medicine. Unlike many herbal medicines, garlic has held up well to scientific investigations. Among documented effects, garlic inhibits bacterial and fungal infections, lowers blood cholesterol, and reduces the risk of stomach cancer.

Garlic forms a bulb, normally comprised of a cluster of 5 to 20 cloves. It is propagated by planting the cloves individually. Garlic prefers a light loam soil and does not compete well with weeds. Frequent shallow weeding or mulch will increase yield. It is susceptible to soil acidity.

As with onion, the green leaves provide the garlic grower with a bonus vegetable. The leaves will have greater nutritional value for the same weight, especially of vitamin A. They contain most of the compounds that give garlic its characteristic flavor and its medicinal properties. Garlic leaves are easy to dry, and powdered garlic leaves make an excellent addition to the kitchen spice rack. Combining garlic leaf and bulb harvest is one of the productive food strategies waiting for more experimentation. The scape, or seed shoot, of both onions and garlic can be eaten like a leaf vegetable as well.

Okra (Abelmoschus esculentus or Hibiscus esculentus)
West African Okra (Abelmoschus caillei)

Okra is an annual member of the hibiscus family. Originally from West Africa, it came to the Western Hemisphere with the slave trade and has now established itself in many of the world's tropical and sub-tropical regions. Okra is particularly popular in West Africa, India, the Philippines, Thailand, and Brazil. It is almost always grown primarily for its mild-flavored, famously mucilaginous immature fruit. However, the use of okra leaves as a potherb is fairly common.

The plant is very tolerant of heat and drought and is rarely damaged by insect pests. It adapts to different soils but the ideal is a slightly acidic, well-drained, sandy soil with plenty of organic matter. Okra usually will thrive as long as it gets full sunlight and adequate water in its first few weeks, but it is a tropical plant that won't tolerate frost. In Africa, growers tend to prefer common okra in dry areas and the large-leafed and quite beautiful West African okra in wetter climates.

Okra seed has a tough coat and will germinate much better if it is soaked overnight before planting. It needs warm conditions for good germination and early growth. Seeds can be planted ½-inch deep three inches apart in rows and thinned two or three times as they begin to crowd each other. The thinnings can be eaten in soups or stews.

The okra plant defends itself by covering all of its parts with tiny hairs, or trichomes, that contain enzymes that can irritate the skin of some people. About one-third of all gardeners are sensitive to these enzymes and do well to wear gloves and long-sleeved shirts when working with okra plants. It is helpful to plant single rows of okra so you can avoid reaching across plants to harvest. Brief

Okra,
*Abelmoschus
esculentus,*
or common okra

cooking eliminates these harmless but slightly irritating trichomes in both the pods and the leaves.

When growing okra for its edible leaves, it can be planted more densely and the leaves continually harvested as they compete for space. The most attractive strategy for gardeners and small subsistence farmers, however, may be to plant seeds at proper spacing for full plants and then partially harvest the leaves for potherbs but not so aggressively that pod formation is prevented. As with many multi-purpose crops, a harvest schedule can favor either leaf or fruit, and developing an optimal combination of leaf and fruit harvests will require some experimentation. If done carefully, partial leaf harvesting may delay fruit harvesting somewhat without significantly lowering the yield. The total yield of protein and most other nutrients will always be higher from a combination leaf and fruit harvest than from harvesting only okra fruits.

Okra leaves are a bit coarser than spinach but can be used in most any recipe calling for greens. They have a slightly tangy flavor from oxalic acid and are often used to thicken soups and stews. Okra leaves can be dried and powdered for use as a nutritious thickening agent. They are extraordinarily rich in calcium and could be a useful vegetable source of this nutrient for people who avoid dairy products. Okra is a thrifty, self-reliant plant with edible pods and leaves, and as if that were not enough, it has dazzling yellow to reddish flowers.

Onion (Allium cepa)

Onions are a nearly universal cool-season crop, but they are originally from Central Asia. They can be started from seeds, sets, or bulbs. Onions and garlic are members of the lily family. Although there are several perennial members of the onion family, the common bulb onion is a biennial almost always grown as an annual. The onion bulb is actually comprised of the swollen bases of leaves. Above the bulb, three to eight leaf blades form. They are hollow and grow nearly vertically.

Dry and cool conditions favor optimal growth of both leaves and bulbs. Onions grow well on soil pH from 5.6 to 7.0, but abundant soil calcium is needed to improve disease tolerance. Rotating the location of onion planting every year helps prevent common fungal diseases. Usually the best-quality and longest-keeping onion bulbs are obtained by planting seed, but crops

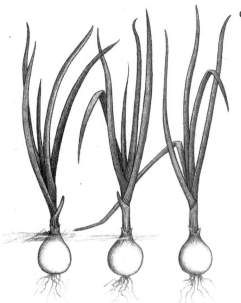

Onion and Garlic,
Allium cepa and
A. sativum

can develop several weeks faster if you plant sets or tiny bulbs. Onions have shallow roots and compete poorly with weeds. For this reason, frequent shallow cultivation or a layer of mulch is beneficial.

After five hollow leaves have formed, some leaves can be snipped off to use as greens with little damage to bulb production. There is no sure formula for knowing how much leaf can be harvested before bulb yield declines unacceptably. It is relatively easy to experiment with two or three small onion patches to get a feel for it. The total yield of useful vegetables from combining partial leaf harvest with bulb harvest will always exceed bulb yield alone. Cut the leaves cleanly rather than tearing them off in order to minimize bacterial or fungal problems.

Leftover onion sets can be planted densely in containers to provide a nearly continual supply of onion leaves for flavoring dishes or to spice up salads. Any surplus of onion leaves can be easily dried and later used as flakes or powder to add to sauces and other dishes. Some West African cultures cut all the leaves that are still green at bulb harvest and pound them into a pulp that is then fermented and sun-dried for use later in seasoning stews and soups. Drying the leaves quickly but out of sunlight will preserve much more of the beta-carotene.

Recognizing the value of the onion's green leaves increases the already impressive culinary adaptability of this vegetable. They are an excellent source of vitamin A and supply roughly twice the calcium, iron, vitamin C, and folate as an equal weight of onion bulbs. Onion leaves stimulate the body's production of glutathione, a key cancer-fighting antioxidant.

Peppers, Bell and Chili (Capsicum annuum)

Capsicum annuum is a plant species with a huge variety of fruits—ranging from the sweet and bland to fiery hot—that evolved between southern Mexico and the Amazon region. Bell or sweet peppers are mild-flavored vegetables used in salads and a variety of cooked dishes, including stuffed peppers. Sweet pepper is eaten in large enough quantities to be considered a vegetable, while the spicier peppers are eaten in smaller quantities as a condiment or spice.

All the peppers are heat-loving, frost-sensitive plants. They can be grown in partial shade, though this may delay fruit formation. They prefer slightly acid, well-drained soils and are somewhat sensitive to waterlogging and to soil salinity.

The young pepper leaves can be used in soups and stews. Leaves should be lightly pruned with a sharp knife or scissors after the plant is at least three weeks old. A chicken stew called *tinola* in the Philippines is probably the most famous dish employing pepper leaves. Only modest amounts of pepper leaf should be eaten, as they contain two mildly toxic compounds.

Radish (Raphanus sativus)

Radishes are annuals in the mustard family, usually grown for their edible swollen roots, though some varieties are used for fodder and cover crops. They originated in the area around the Caspian Sea, and spread rapidly along trade routes. Radishes are now grown nearly worldwide, though they favor cooler locations. They range from the size of a small marble to that of a basketball, and their shape varies from long and slender to spherical. Small radishes can be sown at the first sign of spring and harvested three to five weeks later. The larger Asian varieties usually take about eight to ten weeks from sowing till harvesting. Radishes must grow rapidly with abundant soil moisture or the roots can become tough and harsh flavored. They are sometimes interplanted with lettuce or carrots.

Smaller radishes are usually eaten raw, while the larger ones may be stir-fried or used in soups. They all share the characteristic sharp flavor of horseradish and mustard, derived mainly from sulfur-bearing compounds called glucosinolates. These are primary cancer-fighting phytochemicals, which give radishes a potentially important role in preventive health care.

Though not nearly as popular as beet or turnip greens, the leaves of radishes make a passable potherb. The raw leaves are a bit furry, but even brief cooking eliminates the leaf hairs, or trichomes. One of the good things about radishes as a multi-use crop is that there is little conflict between the use of the leaves and the yield of the roots. Because the roots are grown more for crispness than maximum size, the leaves can just be harvested together with the roots, and then prepared separately. Radish leaves have about six times more vitamin C than the roots, and substantially higher levels of vitamin A, folate, calcium, and protein.

Squash or Cucurbit family
Summer Squash, Winter Squash, Pumpkins, Gourds (Cucurbita pepo)
Winter Squash, Pumpkins (Cucurbita mixta, C. maxima, C. moschata),
Chayote (Sechium edule)
Bottle Gourd (Lagenaria siceraria)
Bitter Gourd (Momordica charantia)
Loofah (Luffa aegyptiaca)

The squash, or Cucurbitaceae, family has over 800 species originating primarily in Central and South America and secondarily in tropical Asia and Africa. They have been useful to humans both as food and as vessels for at least 10,000 years. Hard-shelled gourds, along with coconuts, can stay afloat for months and thus were among the few food plants to have spread across the oceans without human assistance.

Most cucurbits are annuals that use tendrils to climb whatever nearby structure or plant is handy. Some, like pumpkins, have more of a low, sprawling habit. A few varieties of edible squash have even been bred for the plant to have a compact upright bush form. Although tropical in origin, many members of the squash family are quite well adapted to the temperate zone, though none tolerate frost. They grow best with temperatures between 77–86°F and should not be planted until the soil is thoroughly warmed in the spring.

All of the squashes and gourds are heavy feeders that thrive in rich, well-drained soil. Most do best with about one inch of water a week. There are several important pests of the cucurbit family. These include squash vine borers, which are the larvae of small gray moths that infest the stems of squash plants, cucumber beetles, and squash bugs. If the plants can be protected with floating row covers until they begin flowering, most of the insect problems can be avoided. It

Chayote,
Sechium edule

is difficult to keep climbing plants covered that long, but even a couple of weeks of early protection will minimize insect damage. Sometimes, moving the sowing date of cucurbits up or back by a week or two will reduce the intensity of insect attacks.

Cucurbits are grown for a variety of useful products. Immature fruits, such as cucumbers and zucchini, and mature fruits, such as pumpkins and butternut squash, are the most familiar. The hard-shelled gourds are used for ornaments, as containers of all sorts, and even as resonators on stringed instruments. Loofahs (*Luffa aegyptiaca*) are valued for the strong sponge-like fiber inside mature fruits, and are used for scrubbers and in filters. Their immature fruits are eaten like zucchinis in much of Asia. Many cucurbit seeds are roasted and eaten as snacks, and pumpkin seeds are a well-known and commercially marketed food. All of the seeds of this family are rich in oil and protein.

What is not well known, especially in North America, is that the leaves of most cucurbit plants are edible and nutritious. Many Asian and African cultures value the leaves of fluted pumpkin, ivy gourd, chayote, oyster nut, and bitter gourd among others, and these can sometimes be found in local markets. They are almost always cooked and typically prepared in soups or sauces that add flavor, vitamins, and minerals to bland starchy staple foods, especially rice, corn, sorghum, millet, and cassava. Generally, pumpkin leaves are not exactly delicious, but neither are they unpalatable. The flavor of bitter gourd leaves on the other hand are, as the name would suggest, very bitter. Leaves that are bitter or mucilaginous are sometimes greatly valued in African and Asian cuisines.

There are several ways to produce edible leaves from the squash family. Plants grown just for leaves can be sown much more densely than when grown for the fruits. Alternatively, they can be planted densely and repeatedly thinned until they reach a good plant density for growing pumpkins or squash, usually about 4 feet apart. In this case, the thinnings are eaten for greens, leaving space for the few remaining plants to mature. This strategy works best when seed is cheap or plentiful—and especially if you save your own seeds.

Plants can also be grown as they normally would be for fruits, with some limited harvesting of leaves. Light, partial leaf harvest usually won't depress the yield of fruit. Another technique is to plant leftover seed late in the season when there is not sufficient time for fruit to form but there is still plenty of growing season for a good crop of leaves.

Oyster nut (*Telfairia pedata*) and ivy gourd (*Coccinia grandis*) are perennial members of the pumpkin family with edible leaves. They stand apart because they can actually become troublesome invasive plants in the tropics. They should be planted with great caution if at all, and not be introduced into areas where they are not already grown.

Turnips (Brassica rapa *var.* rapa)

Turnips are members of the mustard family that have long been used for both food and fodder, and, as described in Chapter 11, as a cover crop. Turnips are an ancient crop that traveled with Alexander the Great on his conquests. The Irish used them as jack-o-lanterns long before Americans replaced them with pumpkins for Halloween. They are one of the easiest of all crops to grow and they thrive in most climates and soil types.

Turnips are really two nutritious vegetables in one: the smooth white or purple-topped roots and the leafy green tops. While some cultivars such as Shogoin are grown mainly as a leaf crop, and others, like Purple Top, are grown mainly for roots, most turnip varieties will produce good yields of both. In most of the US they can be sown in early spring or in late summer for a fall crop. Seed is usually cheap, so it is feasible to broadcast turnips and thin them as they begin crowding each other, or to grow them as a cover crop.

Thinnings make excellent greens. While partial harvesting of leaves can somewhat reduce the yield of roots, turnips are such a productive, low-maintenance crop that an abundant harvest of both greens and roots is within the reach of even novice gardeners.

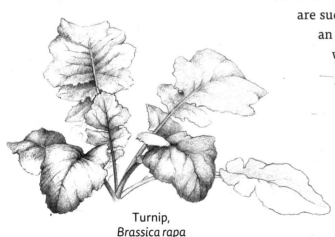

Turnip,
Brassica rapa

Both parts of the turnip are nutritious vegetables, but again, the green leaves outperform the roots. Turnip greens are one of the best sources of the beta-carotene that is converted to vitamin A, while the roots lack this nutrient. Compared to the roots, turnip greens also have three times the iron and vitamin C, six times the calcium, and 13 times the folate.

Other Crops with Edible Leaves As a Secondary Product

Cockscomb (Celosia cristata *or* Celosia argentea *var.* cristata)

A very popular home garden plant usually grown for its tight clusters of brilliant reddish purple flowers, cockscomb is closely related to quail grass and it too has edible and nutritious leaves. It is an easy-to-grow, heat-loving plant that prefers full sunlight but will get along in partial shade. It is prone to fungal disease in poorly drained soil. Cockscomb leaves can be partially harvested about 40 days after planting, and the leaves can be harvested at least twice before the plant is allowed to flower. Leaves are tender and mild flavored. They are best when steamed or boiled, then rinsed. Pinching the earliest flower buds will encourage more flowers to develop on side branches. Once flowering is underway, the leaves become more fibrous.

Grapes (Vitis vinifera)

One of the oldest cultivated crops, grapes have been grown in the Near East for over 8,000 years. They are now grown throughout the world's temperate zones, with China, the US, Mediterranean Europe, and Chile being the largest producers. Most grapes are from the European species *Vitis vinifera*. Three other species are sometimes used for grapes and for edible grape leaves: *Vitis labrusca*, the North American Concord type grape; *Vitis rotundifolia*, the muscadines; and *Vitis riparia*, the wild grape vine of North America. Grapes are an excellent multi-purpose perennial food crop. About 70 percent of grapes are grown for wine. Fresh table grapes make up most of the remainder, with about three percent grown for raisins, grape juice, and jelly. The leaves are used in several ways, including as wrappers for making dolmas, the famous Mediterranean stuffed grape leaf dish.

Grape Leaves, *Vitis vinifera*

Grape leaves are an extremely good source of beta-carotene, the precursor of vitamin A. They have more than 50 times the vitamin A activity of lettuce or cabbage, the world's two most popular leaf vegetables. In addition, grapes are famously an excellent source of resveratrol, a powerful disease-fighting antioxidant, and the leaves of the grape plant are even richer in resveratrol than the fruit.

Young grape plants can sometimes be bought at farm supply stores. They usually have their root ball wrapped in cloth or plastic. Remove the cloth or plastic and plant in a hole roughly twice the size of the root ball, and then water thoroughly. Grape plants can also be started from cuttings of hardwood from an older grape plant. Cuttings should be 8–16 inches long and taken when there are no leaves on the plant. Push the cuttings into moist sand or potting soil and keep them warm until roots start to develop. Plants are usually set 6 to 10 feet apart to allow room for growth and for air movement.

Grapes prefer to grow in full sunlight. They are very cold hardy but are prone to fungus infections in hot, humid weather. They prefer a well-drained slightly acidic soil. They can be planted more closely together if grown mainly for leaves. Very fertile soil will produce plenty of leaves but not much fruit. Grapes need full sunlight and high temperatures to ripen fruit, but grape leaves can produce abundantly in somewhat cooler and shadier conditions.

Grape plants are normally grown on trellises or fences. Typically, the production of grapes involves pruning a lot of stem and leaf to make way for new growth. The leaves removed by pruning can be used for stuffed grape leaves or dried and used later as a good source of vitamin A and other nutrients. Medium-sized leaves are best for making stuffed grape leaves. Tender young leaves tear, and older leaves may be too tough. Any of them are fine for drying and grinding.

If you are getting grape leaves from someone else, be aware that toxic sprays are sometimes used on grape plants. People rarely consider that the leaves might be harvested and eaten. Don't eat leaves that have been recently sprayed with insecticides or fungicides.

Nasturtium (Tropaeolum majus)

Originally from the foothills of the Andes Mountains in Peru, nasturtium has become well known as a garden flower throughout much of the world. They grow as a somewhat sprawling vine and are easily recognized by their bright orange-yellow or red flowers.

Nasturtiums are easy to grow by direct sowing of the seed after the danger of a frost has passed. They prefer well-drained soil, but excessive nitrogen will result in lots of foliage and few blooms. Some varieties can be trained to climb trellises but they need help because they don't produce tendrils.

They are sometimes considered a good companion plant because of their reputation for repelling insect pests. However, the evidence for this is scant.

Nasturtium leaves, flowers, and buds were eaten by the Incas; after being introduced in Europe, they were used to prevent scurvy. The leaves are a good source of vitamin C, so this was not an imaginary value. The dried seeds were occasionally ground as a substitute for expensive pepper. The leaves are rich in calcium but also quite high in oxalic acid, which somewhat diminishes the bio-availability of the calcium.

Quail Grass, Prince of Wales Feathers, Soko, Lagos Spinach, Nigerian Spinach (Celosia argentea or Celosia plumosa)

Often grown as a flower in North America for its long-lasting pink to purple plumes flower, this annual in the amaranth family is originally from Africa. In addition to being a popular ornamental plant, it is widely grown for its tasty leaves, which are eaten as a nutritious potherb in much of Africa and parts of Asia. It is especially popular as a vegetable in West Africa, where half-kilo bundles of leaves are often sold in the markets.

As a vegetable, it is most often called quail grass or soko. It prefers a soil rich in organic matter. Like amaranth, it is frost sensitive and grows poorly at temperatures below 68°F. It will thrive in full sunlight or in partial shade. Once established, quail grass will usually produce plenty of healthy volunteer seedlings that can be harvested as baby greens or transplanted for better yield and easier management. The transplants can be set at about 6 inches apart in all directions. The plants can be uprooted four weeks after transplanting, or pruned to encourage growth of side shoots. Four or five harvests can usually be made at two-week intervals before flowering begins. Quail grass is less bothered by insects than amaranth.

Quail grass is always cooked, and the flavor is better when it is rinsed after boiling. It is a good source of iron, vitamin A, and vitamin C. Unfortunately, oxalic acid reduces the nutritional value of the minerals in quail grass. Preliminary tests with the leaves and the seeds of quail grass have shown some promising anti-viral properties as well

Quail Grass,
Celosia argentea

as a potential lowering of blood sugar. It is extremely easy to grow, nutritious, and a very attractive plant.

Roselle (Hibiscus sabdariffa)

Roselle, or Jamaican sorrel as it is sometimes called, is an annual herb in the hibiscus family, probably originating in southeast Asia. It can grow to 9 feet tall but is usually pruned to keep it shorter and bushier. It is an attractive plant with dark green leaves and purple stems and flowers. It is most often grown for the deep red-colored calyx, or flower bud. These are used to flavor and color sauces, syrups, jams, and for especially refreshing teas and sweetened drinks. The young leaves of the roselle are sometimes eaten raw in salads or added to stir-fried dishes. They are moderately rich in vitamins A and C, calcium, magnesium, and iron.

Roselle can be started from seeds or from stem cuttings. Plants started from seed tend to be somewhat hardier. It grows best in full sunlight but can tolerate some shade. Roselle is not too picky about soil but cannot tolerate waterlogging or frost. It is little bothered by pests. Leaves can be harvested two or three times, beginning about 45–60 days after planting. Calyces can be harvested several times, beginning 80–120 days after planting.

Roselle,
Hibiscus sabdariffa

Spiderplant, Cat's Whiskers, Spider Flower (Cleome gynandra)

Spiderplant, or cat's whiskers, is a popular annual flower growing up to 60 inches tall. It probably originated in south Asia, but is now grown as a vegetable and as an ornamental throughout the world. Although rarely eaten in North America, the young leaves of this plant are especially popular as a potherb in southern Africa, where it is sometimes called African cabbage.

Spiderplant prefers soil that is slightly acid, well-drained and relatively rich in organic matter. It won't tolerate frost and doesn't grow well below 60°F. Because it uses the C4 photosynthetic system, spiderplant thrives on intense sunlight and high temperature and is not very shade tolerant.

Spiderplant is usually grown in rows spaced 12–24 inches apart. Seeds germinate in four to eight days. Three weeks later, they can be thinned to about 4–8 inches between the plants. It is often grown from volunteers that can be transplanted when they are very young to achieve optimal spacing. Spiderplant is slightly prone to powdery mildew and is frequently attacked by aphids, flea beetles, harlequin bugs, and nematodes. On the other hand, it repels some insects and has been intercropped with beans and cabbage family plants to reduce the damage they suffer from diamondback moth larvae and thrips.

Leaves are usually harvested by pruning the growing tips every two weeks. This encourages more side shoots and increases the total yield. Harvest can be extended by supplying plentiful water and shading the plants. Older leaves develop a strong bitter flavor, so harvest only young leaves. With careful management, a yield of seven pounds in ten square feet of garden bed is feasible.

Spiderplant leaves are rich in protein, iron, and calcium. In Africa, they are often cooked with milk or peanuts, or mixed with milder-flavored greens to make the flavor more appealing. The leaves are frequently dried for later use when fresh leaves are hard to find. Spiderplant is very easy to grow, has attractive flowers, and is an excellent source of dietary iron.

Wolfberry, Goji Berry, Chinese Boxthorn, Matrimony Vine (Lycium barbarum, Lycium chinense)

Wolfberry or goji berry are common names given to two closely related perennial members of the large nightshade family, which also includes potatoes, tomatoes, eggplants, and peppers, as well as petunias and tobacco. Both are native to China, where they grow wild and where they have also been cultivated for centuries. With bright green foliage, red or pink flowers, and scarlet berries, wolfberry plants were attractive enough to be imported as ornamentals into Europe.

Although sometimes grown as ornamentals, in their native Asia they are more often valued for the health-giving properties of both the leaves and the berries. Wolfberry plants are mentioned for their health-promoting qualities in a seventh-century Chinese medicinal text. The fruit has recently been added to the growing list of "miracle foods" by aggressive marketers in the West, who often call it Tibetan or Himalayan Goji berry. The berries are very rich in vitamin C and antioxidants, but clinical studies have shown little in the way of miracles. On the other hand, wolfberry *leaves* are an extraordinary source of dietary iron. In extensive testing at the Asian Vegetable Research and Development Center in Taiwan, wolfberry had by far the highest content of iron among vegetable crops.

Wolfberry plants are quite variable in form, ranging up to ten feet tall. They can quickly generate rambling new plants from root suckers. Stems can also form new plants when bent over enough to come into contact with the soil. Some care needs to be taken to keep wolfberry from spreading from its original location in your garden. Plants are usually propagated from stem cuttings or re-rooting suckers, but they also produce viable seed. Eight-inch-long pieces of hardwood stem can be started in the spring or fall. Waiting to harvest leaves until the plant is well established will lead to a longer harvest period. Wolfberry will gradually lose its vigor and is usually replanted every four or five years.

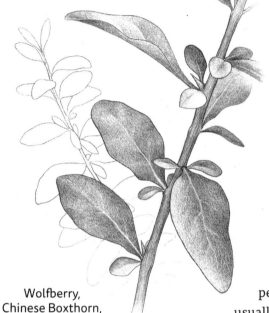

Wolfberry,
Chinese Boxthorn,
Goji Berry,
Lycium barbarum
and *L. chinense*

It is a cold hardy plant but benefits from heavy mulch in hard winter areas. It can also be grown as a container plant and brought inside to winter over until milder weather. It will survive in most conditions but produces more greens and fruit if given good drainage and plenty of organic matter. It is somewhat prone to powdery mildew.

Wolfberry is a true multi-purpose crop, providing both valuable leafy greens and fruit. Frequent trimming of leaves and stems keeps it orderly and very productive. Wolfberry is often grown as a dense hedge in China. In Asia, the leaves are most often stripped from the stem (carefully, to avoid thorns) and stir-fried, steamed, or added to soups. Wolfberry leaves have a somewhat bitter flavor, though it is a flavor that is often appreciated in China.

There are many other plants that have edible leaves as secondary products. Of special importance are the leaves of the tropical staple crops cassava

(*Manihot esculenta*); taro (*Colocasia esculenta*); and malanga (*Xanthosoma sagittifolium*). Because this book is oriented toward temperate-zone gardeners who typically wouldn't have growing seasons that are long enough to produce these starchy underground staples, instructions on growing them have not been included. However, taioba, as the leaves of malanga are called, was included in Chapter 7 because it can be grown strictly as a leaf crop in much of the temperate zone.

9

Two Seasons for Every Purpose Under Heaven?

❊ ❊ ❊

Growing Fresh Greens Year-Round

Humans require a lot of food. We are big, warm-blooded, and active, and our large brains require an extra ration of food to remember pop song lyrics or where the car keys were left. Pound for pound cold-blooded animals, such as alligators, only need about one-tenth as much food as us because they don't need to keep burning food to stay warm. Warm-blooded bears the size of humans often hibernate to save the expense of food over the winter months when it is hardest to come by. Dolphins, whales, and seals are warm-blooded, but are buoyed by the water so they don't need to use fuel in order to stay standing upright. Lions just lounge around for days on end when they are not hunting. No jogging or racquetball.

All that food we need starts out when sunlight hits green leaves and photosynthesis makes sugar. It happens between 32 and 98°F. The rate of photosynthesis generally increases as the temperature warms, reaching peak efficiency at around 77°F. After that, efficiency reaches a plateau, gradually declining until about 98°F, when photosynthesis stops.

Cold weather is hard on plants. They can't move to seek shelter the way animals do. Temperatures below the freezing point of water not only stop photosynthesis, they quickly kill many plants. When water within and between the plant cells freezes, sharp ice crystals form that can rupture the cell walls that house the plant's functional components. In freezing weather, plants can die from dehydration because water in its solid form can't be pumped through the vascular system. Membranes that filter and organize plant nutrients become too stiff to do their jobs, and the activity of essential enzymes becomes too slow to be effective.

In addition to sufficient warmth, maximum food production requires about ten hours or more of daily sunlight. About 2.5 billion people live in temperate climates where, for part of the year, the temperature drops below 32°F and where some of the winter days are less than ten hours long.[1] For at least part of the year these folks need food from *somewhere* warmer and sunnier—or food preserved from *sometime* warmer and sunnier. The industrial food system moves food all over the globe and processes it to extend its shelf life. The local food movement is trying to create regional food economies so that we can reduce how much food needs to be brought in to our communities from afar.

Several thousand years ago we began learning how to preserve food so that supplies could be carried forward from times of abundance to times of scarcity. Fattening animals over the summer to slaughter in the fall or winter is part of this tradition. Canning or freezing the surplus from the kitchen garden is another way to bring the products of photosynthesis into the future. Probably the oldest human means of preserving food is drying. Simple techniques for drying leaf crops for year-round use can be found in Chapter 12. In addition to importing food or preserving it, we can sometimes modify the climate of small spaces to favor photosynthesis.

How difficult it is to create a microclimate for winter vegetable growing depends mainly on where you are and what you are trying to grow. The map shows the US Department of Agriculture Plant Hardiness Zones. The zones range from 1 to 11, with 1 being frigid polar conditions and 10 and 11 being tropical and frost-free. The average minimum temperature in zone 1 is lower than minus 50°F, while in zone 11 it is above 40°F. Each zone has a minimum temperature roughly 10°F warmer than the zone before it.

The period between the average last frost in the spring and the average first frost in the fall is called the growing season. In zones 1 and 2, the growing season is less than 90 days, while in zone 10 the growing season is 365 days a year. In the US and southern Canada, most people live in zones 3–8. The longer your growing season, the less you need to modify your climate in order to produce food year round.

A few things jump out at you looking at the zone map. The most obvious is that it gets colder as you move further away from the equator. As a very rough rule of thumb, temperature drops about three degrees Fahrenheit for every 300 miles you move away from the equator. This is only true at sea level.

The second thing you may notice on the plant hardiness zone map is that temperatures tend to be milder near the coasts and colder further inland. Coastal parts of the northern states of Maine and Washington have roughly the same length growing season as Kentucky, Missouri, and Kansas far to the south. This is largely due to the *thermal flywheel effect* of trillions of gallons of seawater. The water absorbs heat over the summer and then gradually releases it over the winter. This has the effect of making the summers a little cooler and the winters a bit warmer. This moderating impact on climate is part of the reason why roughly half of the world's population resides within 60 miles of a coastline.

More astute students of geography may notice that much of the Rocky Mountain area has a colder climate and a shorter grower season than surrounding areas at the same latitude. Another very rough rule of thumb is that the temperature drops three and a half degrees Fahrenheit for every 1,000 foot increase in elevation. So at 6,000 feet, you could expect it to be 21 degrees cooler than at sea level.

In order to photosynthesize and make food, plants need a minimum of both sunlight and warmth. Summer tends to have both. Most of the temperate zone gets about half of its total annual allotment of solar energy over 100 summer days. However, the research of Maine winter gardener, Eliot Coleman, has shown that as long as there are ten hours or more of daylight, there is still enough light intensity to produce food for most of the rest of the year.[2] Everything south of the 32nd parallel gets at least ten hours of daylight all year round. As you move north, the number of days with less than ten hours of sunshine increases. New York City has about 68 days a year that fall short of ten hours of daylight. By Montreal, that number has risen to 90 days, and by Winnipeg on the 50th parallel there are 106 days with too little daylight for good plant growth.

In practice, this means that you should time the planting of winter crops so they can make the most of their growth by the time day length falls below ten hours. If the temperature doesn't get much below freezing, most cold hardy crops can be kept in a state of healthy dormancy or slow growth through this period of sub-optimal day length. In other words, you won't be

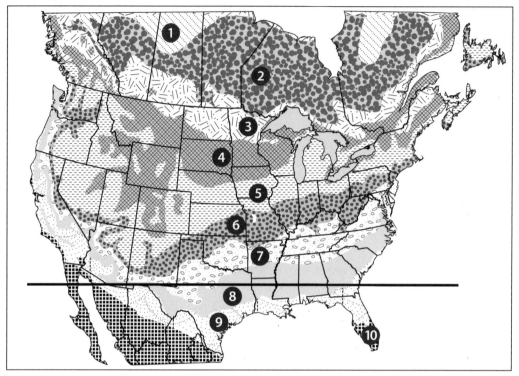

USDA Plant Hardiness Zones with an approximation of the 32nd parallel

Starlight, Star Bright?

We look to the sky and see the moon and the stars. The nearest star, our sun, delivers about half a million times more energy per square meter than the moon and about 80 million times more energy than the more distant visible stars. Here is a listing of the approximate intensity of light from natural sources, in watts, hitting a square meter of surface:

Starlight: 0.000002 watts

Moonlight: 0.000322 watts

Overcast daylight: 16.1 watts

Direct sunlight: 161.0 watts

Source: Smith, Shane (2000) *Greenhouse Gardener's Companion, Revised: Growing Food & Flowers in Your Greenhouse or Sunspace*, Colorado: Fulcrum Publishing, page 15.

producing a great deal of new food but you can still harvest fresh vegetables. While you can't do much about the tilt of the Earth, you can make the most out of the available sunlight by minimizing shadows and using reflective surfaces to bounce additional light onto plants.

Sunlight is a relatively fixed input, but the innovative gardener can still take two long strides toward growing fresh food during cold weather. The first, and probably most obvious, is to plant cold-hardy vegetable crops. The second is to create miniature spaces with slightly modified climates that favor the growth of plants.

Cold-Hardy Crops

Some food crop species are much more resistant to cold than others. How do kale and turnips fend off temperatures below freezing, and why are tomatoes or sweet potatoes or pole beans unable to do the same? Cold-hardy plants have at least two slightly different strategies for preventing fatal ice crystal formation. The most common approach is to lower the freezing point of the water they hold with dissolved sugars and the amino acid, proline. This is akin to putting salt on icy roads to lower the temperature at which the water freezes. The second and more amazing trick of cold-hardy crops is the use of "antifreeze" proteins, or ice-structuring proteins. These are specialist protein molecules that some plants are able to make. They bind to the surface of tiny ice crystals and prevent them from forming the large and sharp crystals that rupture plant cells.

Why can't peppers, zucchini, and tomatoes use these same tricks? Because they evolved in warm regions; they didn't need to outwit winter. Plants—or animals for that matter—will rarely invest the resources to develop an ability that has no survival value.

Cold-hardy vegetable crops are generally plants that can thrive in low light levels as well as low temperatures. They are plants that don't need a long growing season, and generally these plants are not grown for their fruit. They are most often leaf crops that have some degree of genetic tolerance for cold weather and limited sunlight.[3] Master winter vegetable grower Eliott Coleman lists 30 crops he has grown successfully over the winter in Maine. They are: arugula, beet greens, broccoli raab, carrots, chard, chicory, claytonia, collards, dandelion, endive, escarole, garlic greens, kale, kohlrabi, leeks, lettuce, mache, minutina, mizuna, mustard greens, pak choi, parsley, radicchio, radish, scallions, sorrel, spinach, tatsoi, turnips, and watercress.

Of these, carrots and radish are root crops; kohlrabi is grown for its swollen stem; and the other 27 are leaf crops.[4] Among those 27 crops you can find tasty, nutritious, and easy-to-grow varieties to fill your winter vegetable garden.

Microclimate Change for Cold Weather

Choosing vegetable crops that have genetically adapted to cold weather moves you in the direction of fresh food all winter long. Growing those plants in microclimates that have been modified to be a bit warmer can get you the rest of the way. The most cost-effective approach is usually to simply raise winter temperatures a few degrees so that cold hardy vegetables can be grown later than is normally possible. Raising the winter temperature a few degrees for some of your garden plants is akin to moving them into a hardiness zone with a slightly longer growing season.

The simplest approach is looking for warmer microclimates in your garden. Land sloping to the south or west will often pick up enough extra sunshine to extend growing temperatures for a week a so. A wall to the north or east will trap some extra heat for nearby plants and block out cold, dry winds, which reduces stress on winter vegetable crops. Depressions or sunken spots in the garden are usually poor choices for winter vegetables because cold air is heavier than warm air and will drain into low areas.

For more winter protection, you need to enclose plants in some way so that heat is not instantly lost to the colder surroundings. When you enclose plants, it is essential that at least part of the covering facing south allows enough light to pass through to drive photosynthesis. Four basic questions need to be answered before successfully growing enclosed winter crops:

- How big will the enclosure be?
- What material will allow the sunlight to pass into the enclosure?
- How will the enclosure be heated?
- How can the heat be retained?

How Big?

People have grown winter greens in every imaginable size of enclosure, from cloches (individual plant covers) to gigantic greenhouses. In between are cold frames, low tunnels, and high tunnels (hoop houses). Cold frames are small enclosures that may be covered by a couple of old window sashes or other transparent material. Low tunnels are usually clear polyethylene sheeting over hoops that may cover whole rows or beds of plants. High tunnels, also called hoop houses, usually cover several beds and are tall enough to walk into. Greenhouses are generally more permanent structures that can range from tiny to huge. They can be free-standing, attached to a building, or dug into the ground. Obviously, larger enclosures can produce more greens, but unless you are selling them, it is easy to grow more than you need.

Rapidly fluctuating temperatures are very hard on plants. Because temperatures in the natural world rarely change dramatically over a short time, few plants have evolved mechanisms to adapt to rapid fluctuations. Smaller enclosures are far more prone to fluctuating temperatures than larger ones. The temperature inside cloches and small cold frames can go from near freezing on a cold morning to 100 degrees before noon if there is a clear sky. They overheat quickly in full sunlight and cool just as quickly when the sun stops shining.

Growing enclosures need to be vented to allow excess heat to escape, and this is often impractical with very small enclosures. Larger cold frames and greenhouses have greater volumes of air and a greater mass of plants and soil, so they take longer to heat up and longer to dissipate their heat when outside temperatures cool. This results in less rapid temperature changes and happier plants. Home gardeners rarely have the space, the money, or the need for a greenhouse large enough for optimal thermodynamics, so they have to make compromises and pay careful attention to venting.

Let in Sunlight

The light-transmitting covering used for plant enclosures is usually called *glazing*; glass has traditionally been the preferred material. More recently, several plastics have become popular for glazing plant-growing enclosures. Which glazing is best depends mainly on the size of the enclosure and the budget for the project. Some of the commonly used glazing materials are compared below. Prices listed are as of October 2013 in US dollars per square foot. They are given here simply to offer an idea of relative cost.

Glass is excellent at allowing sunlight to pass through but it is heavy and relatively expensive. Because of its weight and brittleness, glass is usually not available in large sheets. Piecing together smaller panes of glass can be labor intensive and can result in air leaks and weak spots. Glass is made from sand and is nearly inert chemically, which makes it a very durable material. It can easily outlive its petroleum-based plastic alternatives. On the other hand, glass doesn't coexist well with hailstorms, baseball games, or BB guns. Because it is so clear, it is great for looking through, but it also tends to throw sharp shadows on the plants; a more diffused light is better suited to reaching the lower leaves of plants. Double pane glass holds heat in better than single pane, but is even heavier and more expensive. Used windows and sliding glass doors are frequently available cheaply or for free.

Acrylic is a rigid very clear plastic that is the second most durable common glazing material, usually lasting 20 years or more. It is available in single and double wall panels. As of October 2013, it cost over $3 per square foot. More often used in skylights or sunrooms, acrylic is a rather expensive choice for extending the season for your vegetable garden. It needs to be installed very carefully to avoid cracking or allowing air leaks from expansion and contraction.

Polycarbonate is plastic glazing that is becoming more popular. It usually lasts 12–20 years before discoloring. It comes as single sheets and as double or triple wall sheets with air spaces between the layers. Single sheets cost about $1.20 per square foot, and triple wall costs nearly three times as much. Polycarbonate provides good-quality diffused light for your plants. It is easy to work with and won't break from hail or stray foul balls. On the downside, polycarbonate glazing is still quite expensive, especially the multi-layer sheets, and it scratches easily.

Fiberglass glazing is usually sold as corrugated sheets or in 50-foot-long rolls. Both are about four feet wide. It is tough, has good light transmission, and is reasonably easy to work with. It is often guaranteed for ten years, after which it begins to yellow, and the glass fibers become exposed. It is currently selling for $1.60 to $2.30 per square foot—somewhat less expensive than either acrylic or twin-wall polycarbonate.

Polyethylene sheeting is the lowest cost option for winter glazing. Avoid buying the utility grade polyethylene sheeting available in hardware and building supply stores. It degrades into a mess of plastic chips in a year or less of full sunlight. Get 4-year 6-mil UV-treated greenhouse-grade sheeting. This has become popular for big hoop houses growing tomatoes and greens commercially. Its main advantage is that it is cheap. It's also helpful that it comes in large, lightweight sheets. This allows simple framing with a minimum of joints. The obvious drawback is that it must be replaced more frequently than other glazings. It is fairly tough, but high winds and cats' claws can damage it. The appearance of large polyethylene-covered structures is considered to be a negative factor in many residential settings.

Because poly sheeting is very inexpensive, growers in cold climates often can afford to install two layers separated by an air space for greater insulation. Small fans are used to keep the space between the two layers inflated. Using two layers reduces light intensity somewhat, but the savings in heating may offset that loss. A higher-grade twin-wall polyethylene glazing is also available. The single sheets usually sell for $0.13–0.15 per square foot and last four years. The twin-wall polyethylene costs about $1.80 per square foot, but is much sturdier, provides much better insulation, and is guaranteed for ten years.

Warm Up: The most basic way to raise the temperature in winter food-growing structures is to capture the heat energy in sunshine. The sun's energy in the form of light passes easily through glazing and is absorbed by the plants and the soil, where much of the light energy is converted to heat. This heat radiates from the plants and soil, but because heat waves are much longer than light waves, they don't pass as easily back out through the glazing. Thus energy is trapped, and the temperature rises.

In some situations, it is too cold or too cloudy to capture enough heat from sunlight to warm the plants. More often, sunlight will adequately warm the plants during the day but won't keep them warm enough overnight. This is when some form of supplemental heat is needed.

The ideal place to deliver supplemental heat is usually to the soil below the plants. This way, as the heat rises it warms the plant roots and then the plants before being lost through the glazing. Electrical soil heating cables or heating mats can be used for this purpose, but they can be expensive both to purchase and to operate if you are trying to keep more than a small area warm. They are, however, very good for helping get seeds started, as the ideal germination temperature for many plants is higher than their ideal growing temperature. The advantage of heating cables and mats is that they are usually controlled by thermostats, so they turn on and off automatically as the soil temperature drops or rises.

On a larger scale, some greenhouse growers take advantage of the hot air that collects at the top of the structure on a sunny day. Rather than vent it to cool the plants, they recirculate it through tubes buried in the soil to keep the plants warm overnight.

Heating the *air* rather than the soil with electric, gas, or kerosene heaters is usually too wasteful relative to the value of the vegetables produced.

Perhaps the oldest system for heating the soil for winter vegetable growing is the *hot bed*. A traditional hot bed is basically a cold frame with 16 inches or so of fresh barnyard manure placed under six inches of good garden soil. As bacteria breaks down the manure, it heats up, warming the soil above.

When spring arrives, you have a deep bed filled with a warm, super-rich mix of soil and compost. You can then grow heavy feeders like broccoli, corn, celery, or pumpkins in the bed.

Keeping the Heat: However heat is supplied to your winter growing structure, it will try to escape through the glazing. While the sun is shining, you will likely gain more heat through the glazing than you lose, but during long cloudy stretches and especially on cold nights, the opposite will be true. There are two main strategies for slowing heat loss. The first is to insulate the glazing when it is not letting in sunlight. The second is to capture excess solar heat during the day and release it slowly as the temperature drops overnight. The two strategies are often combined.

Insulating: Insulation is material that slows the inevitable movement of heat from a warmer surface toward a colder one. The greater the temperature difference between the two surfaces the faster the heat flows toward the colder one, and the more valuable insulation is in slowing that heat loss. In smaller growing structures, it is usually easier to insulate by covering the glazing from the outside. This can be as simple as tossing an old blanket over your cold frame at night or covering your glazing with a foam panel. For structures large enough to stand up in, insulation is more often applied from the inside. Sheets of bubble wrap can work for this purpose, as it can be pushed against the glazing and the trapped air inside the many bubbles slows the flow of heat. Foiled-covered bubble wrap, available in building supply stores, is doubly effective because it reflects heat as well as slowing its passage through the glazing.

A solar greenhouse takes advantage of the fact that little useful light enters from the north (the opposite is true in the Southern Hemisphere). Rather than having glazing cover the entire structure, the north wall is opaque and well insulated. This slightly diminishes the amount of light that enters but significantly slows heat loss.

A technique that is rapidly becoming more popular with winter growers is the use of row covers. These are sheets of light fabric, usually polypropylene or polyester, that can be laid directly on top of plants or supported over the plants with hoops. Row covers are available in different weights that offer varying degrees of insulation and protection from freezing. They are permeable, allowing both water and sunlight to pass through. In fact, the lightest row covers allow 85 percent of the sunlight through, in effect acting both as glazing and as insulation. The heavier row covers block more sunlight but offer a few more degrees of frost protection.

Row covers can be used alone outside to cover crops or as an additional layer of protection inside a greenhouse or high tunnel. In the warmer parts of the US, row covers alone might get hardy crops through the winter. In areas with moderate winters, a single layer of glazing should suffice, and in the coldest winters row covers within a greenhouse may be necessary. This is often a cheaper and more flexible way to gain a little mid-winter warmth than using two layers of polyethylene sheeting with air blowing between them. It is easier to manage large billowing row covers inside a greenhouse—where the wind doesn't blow. It takes a bit of practice to get the hang of using row covers, but they are definitely a useful tool for winter vegetable gardeners.

Capturing Excess Heat: Capturing excess heat and then gradually releasing it during colder conditions is a function of the thermal flywheel effect. Some materials, such as stone, concrete, and water can act as *heat sinks*, absorbing large amounts of heat during a sunny day and releasing it slowly overnight. Water is especially good at storing heat energy.

You don't have to move to the coast to make use of the thermal flywheel effect to grow winter vegetables. Putting water, gravel, concrete, or brick in your enclosed winter garden can soften the sharp differences between day and night temperatures. These materials, often called *thermal mass*, can soak up sunshine, removing heat from the air and reducing the danger of plants overheating. When the outside temperature drops, the stored heat migrates away from the mass and warms the plants.

The thermal flywheel effect is also at play whenever we dig down a few feet into the ground. Four or five feet down, the temperature is quite stable year round, despite the huge differences in summer and winter temperatures above ground. You can experience this flywheel effect by going into a cave, or a spring, or even a basement. You will feel warmer in the winter and cooler in the summer.

This is the principle that makes the pit greenhouse a compelling idea. Building a greenhouse over a pit or a trench gives your plants the benefit of the earth's giant thermal flywheel, reducing the damaging daily fluctuations of hot and cold. The depth of the pit is somewhat limited by the low angle of the winter sun. A pit greenhouse that is more than five or six feet deep usually won't get adequate sunlight to all the plants. Be aware that drainage is a critical issue with pit greenhouses. Ones that don't drain well invite plant disease problems.

The main goal here is to reduce rapid temperature changes and keep day and night temperatures from being dramatically different, not to get to a single uniform temperature. In fact, most plants grow best when the temperature during the night is about 10 to 15°F lower than the day temperature. This allows them to use less energy for respiration during the cooler night.

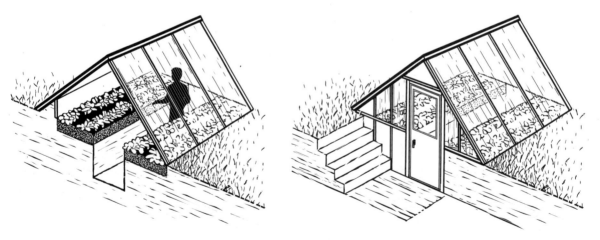

Basic Pit Greenhouse

Fine tuning the type, amount, and placement of thermal mass in a cold frame or small greenhouse is tricky business that rewards both study and experimentation. No matter how carefully you proceed, you shouldn't expect the thermal flywheel to fully resolve all your heating and ventilation problems. It is easy to get intimidated by all the details and calendars and math involved in winter gardening, but the underlying reality is that with just a little bit of help, cold-hardy leafy greens will do the heavy lifting. Most gardeners will succeed.

Too Hot: Growing greens into and through a cold winter is a challenge that most enthusiastic gardeners can rise to, but sometimes we are faced with just the opposite problem. We want to grow greens but it has gotten too hot. Few food plants grow well at temperatures over 90°F. The increasingly long and hot days of summer can cause bolting, or premature flowering. When plants begin to flower, their leaves normally donate protein and sugars to the reproductive process; consequently, the leaves develop harsher flavors and tougher textures.

In much of the US, the spring season for growing greens ends abruptly with the first hot days. This is largely a function of the leaf crops that we have chosen to grow. Lettuce, spinach, cabbage, and the so-called "southern greens" (kale, collards, mustard, and turnip greens) make up over 95 percent of all the greens Americans eat. These are all crops better adapted to cold than to heat.

The same two basic strategies—choosing naturally adapted plants and creating modified microclimates—work equally well in extending the growing season through scorching weather as they do extending it through frigid times. If you decide to go this route, though, you may need to be a bit more adventurous about what is for supper.

Heat-Tolerant Crops

The most effective step toward cultivating hot-weather greens is to grow leaf crops adapted to the tropics. The vast majority of the world's plant species are native to the tropics. Not surprisingly, plants that evolved in tropical lowlands are well adapted to heat. You may live far from the tropics, but even as far north as southern Canada, the climate in July is essentially tropical.

Among tropical plants that can be easily grown for edible leaves in the summer throughout most of North America are: amaranth (*Amaranthus* spp.), cowpeas(*Vigna unguiculata*), cranberry hibiscus (*Hibiscus acetosella*), jute (*Corchorus olitorius*), okra, purslane (*Portulaca oleracea*), quail grass (*Celosia argentea*), roselle (*Hibiscus sabdariffa*), sweet potato, and vine spinach (*Basella alba*). Heat-adapted leaf crops that are somewhat more challenging to grow include chaya (*Cnidoscolus aconitifolius*), moringa (*Moringa oleifera*), Okinawa spinach (*Gynura crepioides*), and toon (*Toona sinensis*).

In most of North America, most of these crops will benefit from being started in a protected environment a few weeks before the soil warms.

Cowpeas (black-eyed peas), okra, and sweet potatoes are well-known garden plants, but they are not normally grown for their edible leaves. When growing these crops primarily for their leaves, they should be planted about twice as densely as usual. The remaining hot-weather leaf crops are somewhat less familiar. They are discussed in Chapter 7.

Some plants, including corn, sorghum, and sugarcane, use the highly efficient C4 photosynthetic process. C4 plants have a significant advantage over the more common C3 plants during hot and dry conditions. They can continue photosynthesizing after the leaf stomata have closed to conserve moisture, and they are able to operate at higher light saturations. Although C4 plants make up only about three percent of all plant species, they are estimated to assimilate 30 percent of all atmospheric carbon captured by plants on land. Among leaf crops, amaranth and purslane use the C4 photosynthetic process.

Microclimate Change for Hot Weather

You don't really need to grow unfamiliar tropical plants to get fresh greens through the heat of the summer. You can often push the heat back a few weeks with just a bit of shade. If you can plant on a north or east slope rather than on a southern or western exposure, greens will enjoy slightly cooler weather. Planting heat-sensitive greens on the north side of taller plants, such as corn or sunflowers, can also allow harvests deeper into the summer than greens growing in full sunlight. Also, the same floating row covers that are used to keep plants warm in January can be used to shade them in July.

Commercially available greenhouse shade cloth can be used to produce tender greens through the heat of summer. Shade cloth is available with a range of shading intensities. A study in Kansas, where summer heat severely limits production of greens from June through August, showed that "high tunnels covered with 40% shade cloth combined with drip irrigation were able to produce good crops of lettuce and Asian greens throughout the summer."[5] Shaded plants will grow more slowly; more than 40 percent shade will lead to spindly plants.

In addition to the options listed above, there are a few other tricks that can help with growing greens in hot weather. Planting in *sunken* growing beds will create slightly cooler conditions. Placing a thick layer of mulch around plants will help to keep the soil temperature down in the hottest months. Water has a moderating effect on temperature, so plants grown close to bodies of water may stay slightly cooler and grow better through the summer heat. Plants that are progressively exposed to hot weather will often survive, whereas plants exposed more suddenly may wilt and die. Transplants can be gradually acclimatized to hot weather in the same manner that fall crops can be hardened off for cold weather.

Plants use evaporative cooling to keep leaf temperatures low enough for efficient photosynthesis. They do this by drawing water up from the soil and then releasing it through *stomata* on the undersides of their leaves. When soil moisture is in short supply, leaves wilt and stop producing. Leaf crops typically need about one inch of rain per week for optimum production. This is about 62 gallons for a 100-square-foot bed.

Another technique that can extend the harvest of greens into hot weather is pruning. While premature flowering (bolting) can be brought on by excessive heat or lack of soil moisture, in many leaf crops flowering can be delayed by pinching off the growing tip (apical meristem) of the plant. This causes formation of side shoots and extends both the length of time that greens can be harvested and the total yield.

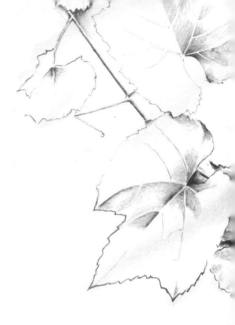

10

Gardening in 3-D

❊ ❊ ❊

Growing Vertical Greens

A constantly replenished wave of light leaves the surface of the sun, races across 93,000,000 miles of swirling space in less than nine minutes and lands on the tender green surface of a living plant. A few trillionths of a second later, the chlorophyll in the leaf has used that photon bit of energy to combine carbon, hydrogen, and oxygen from earth's abundant air and water into sugar, the sweet fuel of life. From this simple sugar are formed complex sugars, starches, and fibers. Plants store the energy from the sunshine in their stems, roots, and fruits. Gardeners and farmers try to manage this biological solar energy collection operation in ways that benefit them. Simply climbing a hill gave me a useful perspective on this important undertaking.

From a hillside overlooking forests and corn fields in late spring, the forest appeared as a plush unbroken carpet of 50 shades of green, while the young corn looked like green lines marked across a sheet of brown paper. Clearly, the forest had more leaves basking in the sunshine than the corn. By late August, the verdant forest was looking down on a cornfield that had already produced all the corn it could and now held lifeless amber waves of grain drying in prime farmland. Yet this cornfield was the culmination of modern agricultural science—dependent on tractors, genetically modified seeds, herbicides, insecticides, and synthetic fertilizers—while the green forest was simply neglected and ignored.

An acre of forest has more surface area of green leaves more of the year than an acre in grain crops. This enables it to produce far more biomass, or living substance. The ratio of the surface area of green leaf to the surface area of the ground below it is called the *Leaf Area Index* (LAI). As a general rule, high LAIs correlate with high net productivity in any terrestrial ecosystem. (Aquatic ecosystems are usually powered by photosynthetic algae rather than leaves.)

Logic would suggest that an LAI above 1.0 is not possible because one square meter of leaf would intercept all of the sunshine falling on one square meter of ground. However, some ecosystems, such as pine forests, actually have LAIs as high as 10. Try reading something in the very shadiest spot in a park or a forest at midday. Despite a seemingly complete cover of tree leaves overhead, your eyes will still intercept enough sunlight to be able to read. Shade isn't darkness. Some of the incoming photons bounce off the leaves back out into space; some pass directly through the thin leaves; and some bounce around until they find your eyes. Logic doesn't appreciate how energetic, quick, and bouncy light energy is.

The ability of green leaves to capture the radiant energy of sunshine and convert it to food and fiber is the basis of life on Earth. The bulk of our food is currently grown in anti-forests: large, uniform plantings of annual grains and soybeans. Most of the advantages of forest over grain fields are a function of greater complexity. Forests have much more diversity of species, of plant sizes and types, and of animal, bacterial, and fungal communities. Complexity increases yield. A very simplistic example of this basic principle can be seen by intercropping corn and cowpeas. Two acres of intercropped corn and cowpeas will typically yield about one-third more than one acre in just corn plus one acre in just cowpeas. Forests extend this principle on every level. The complex interactions among different kinds of living beings in a forest enables more complete harvesting of sunlight and more efficient recycling of nutrients. This complexity not only allows forests to thrive without the fertilizers that drive our food system, it also builds in resilience that monoculture agriculture lacks.

Forests are amazing, but by now you may be wondering if I've overlooked a key point. While forests produce a surprising variety of foods that we could eat, their primary output is the cellulose and lignin in wood. We don't eat wood. A patch of typical North American forest the size of an average home garden (about 600 square feet) would produce a disappointing amount of readily eaten food for a family. However, we can still improve the way we grow much of our food by employing some of the natural advantages that forests have over our grain fields. That is, if we learn to grow in three dimensions instead of two.

The most forest-like plants in the home garden are likely to be dwarf fruit and nut trees. Most tree leaves are too tough to be eaten, but there are a couple of exceptions. In the temperate zone, Chinese toon (*Toona sinensis*) and small-leaved linden (*Tilia cordata*) are two full-sized trees with edible leaves that stand out. In the tropics, moringa (*Moringa oleifera*), and chaya (*Cnidoscolus aconitifolius*) are smaller trees with spectacularly edible leaves. For practical reasons, edible-leafed trees are usually best kept pruned to a height that allows easy leaf harvest.

A Leg Up

The home garden is generally not well suited for making good use of full-size trees, except for shade. However, many of the forest advantages from taller plants and a higher leaf canopy can be simulated by growing climbing plants on trellises. Trellises are frames of any kind that provide support for a climbing or vining plant.

From the point of view of the plant, a trellis offers the opportunity to harvest sunlight above the crowd without the metabolic expense of building a stout trunk. Instead of diverting resources to building its own physical support, the climbing plant can simply attach itself to a trellis and invest more heavily in foliage, roots, transportation of nutrients, and reproduction. For the garden as an ecosystem, trellised plants act as make-shift deciduous trees, providing a wind break, partial shade, and evaporative cooling on hot summer days and losing their leaves to allow the more dilute sunlight of fall, winter, and spring to pass through (to power newly planted cool-weather greens).

From the gardener's perspective, using trellises and climbers allows two to three times greater yield from the same square footage of garden. This allows the gardener to focus resources such as compost and water on a smaller area while harvesting sunshine over a greater area. It is often far easier to keep a few square feet below your trellis weeded, watered, and mulched than to tend to double or triple that area without trellises. Trellised plants also reduce the problem of contamination from soil pathogens splashed up onto leaves by rain. Trellises also provide convenient perches which attract many song birds to serenade the gardener. The birds benefit the garden by eating insects and leaving nutrient-rich droppings.

Most of the leaf vegetables that thrive on trellises are members of the bean and pea family (*Leguminosae*) or members of the pumpkin family (*Cucurbitaceae*). Among climbing legumes, the leaves of peas, common beans, yardlong beans, (*Vigna unguiculata* subsp. *sesquipedalis*), hyacinth beans (*Lablab purpureus*), scarlet runner beans (*Phaseolus coccineus*), rice beans (*Vigna umbellata*), and winged beans (*Psophocarpus tetragonolobus*) are sometimes eaten. Climbing members of the pumpkin family that have edible leaves include chayote (*Sechium edule*), squash, pumpkins, gourds (*Cucurbita pepo*, *C. mixta*, *C. maxima*, *C. moschata*), fluted pumpkin (*Telfaria occidentales*), bitter gourd (*Momordica charantia*), and bottle gourd (*Lagenaria siceraria*). All of these are multi-use plants that are more often grown for their fruit or seed rather than their edible leaves.

Other climbing plants with nutritious leaves that could be more widely eaten include grapes, vine spinach (*Basella alba* and *B. rubra*), and sweet potatoes. Grapes are often used in ornamental horticulture to create shaded arbors, and covered entryways and fences. Vine spinach as its name implies likes to climb whatever is nearby. A perennial in the tropics, it is normally grown as an annual in the warmer parts of the temperate zone. It won't tolerate frost and grows slowly in cool spring weather, but when the weather warms, it wraps around any fence, pole, trellis, or tree and takes off.

Most varieties of sweet potatoes are better described as sprawlers than as climbers. Still, they can be grown over low trellises such as A-frames covered with sturdy fencing. Letting sweet potato plants sprawl over a low trellis helps produce bigger sweet potato yields by preventing the plant from rooting where the vine contacts the soil. These side, or prop, roots can draw energy away from the main root production.

Trellises can be built from a wide variety of materials. Most trellises have a rigid framework to support the weight of the plants and some sort of netting or mesh or fencing that enables the plant to grab hold. I have found cedar poles to make good supports and have nailed hog fencing to the cedar for plant holds. Steel reinforcing mesh for concrete (often called remesh) is another good option for trellises. It has a 6" × 6" steel wire mesh that is strong enough to support any plants, and the openings are large enough to reach through for easy harvesting.

Pre-built trellises can be bought from building supply and garden shops but they are generally expensive and better suited to ornamental landscaping than growing edible leaves. There is some work involved in building good trellises, so it is worth using materials that will hold up for at least a few years. Most people prefer not having pressure-treated wood in their food gardens because of possible leaching of toxic chemicals. Actually, the use of arsenic, by far the most troubling chemical in treated wood, ended in 2003 and was replaced by much safer ACQ (alkaline copper quaternary). While ACQ-treated wood is still not permitted in certified organic production, most experts consider it reasonably safe to use in the garden.

Cedar, locust, cypress, and a few other woods are naturally rot-resistant alternatives to pressure-treated wood, though they can be expensive and hard to find. Building with scrap or used wood and accepting that your wooden trellises will need to be periodically rebuilt is another option.

One of my favorite trellis systems is just six to eight bamboo poles arranged in a tepee. Lay the poles on the ground with the thick end of the bamboos even with each other. Six or seven feet from the bottom, tie them together with a rot-resistant twine and trim off any bamboo more than nine feet long. Then stand them up and spread each individual piece of the base of the bamboo out to make a cone about four feet in diameter and six feet high. (If you are cutting fresh bamboo, don't trim all the side shoots flush. Leaving a bit of side shoot on the bamboo allows climbing plants to take hold easier.) When you cut a stalk of live bamboo, it won't regrow. Lots of people have bamboo patches in their yards that need repeated thinning. They are usually happy to have gardeners do that thinning in exchange for the trellis material.

Any kind of bean or peas or vine spinach planted around the outside of this trellis will happily climb the bamboo. A great arrangement for the bamboo tepee trellis is a donut-shaped bed, made by creating a rim of raised, loosened soil by digging it from out of the center. Then fill the hollow in the center with mulch that will hold moisture and keep weeds from competing with the trellised plants. If you have a patch of bamboo or have neighbors who do, you should always have a supply to make more trellises from thinning the bamboo. They usually need to be replaced every two to three years.

Bamboo trellises are rarely strong enough to support the weight of gourd, pumpkin, and squash plants. Tripods of cedar poles with some cross pieces or heavy fencing work well for these plants. You can easily make a shady spot

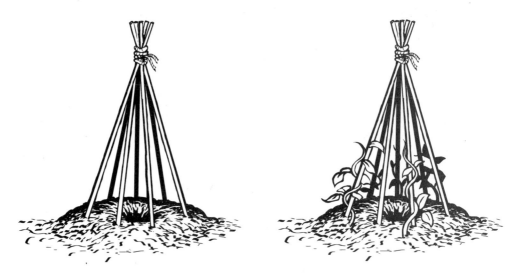

A donut-shaped bed with a bamboo trellis makes good use of space.

for kids to play or to hang a hammock under with these cedar pole trellises. When you add netting or fencing to a trellis, it is helpful to start it 6 inches or so above the ground so that you can easily weed and mulch the young plants. They will find the trellis.

The number of creative ways to build trellises for plants to climb is easily matched by the number of ingenious ways that plants have evolved to climb them. Various plants have modified their stems, branches, leaves, flowers, and even roots to aid in the process of climbing skyward. For example the pumpkin or gourd family (*Cucurbitaceae*) sends out long thin tendrils looking for something to climb. The plants employ a system of hormone controls to elongate the cells on one side of a tendril to move it slowly in a circle until it encounters resistance. When it makes contact, different hormones signal the tendril to wrap tightly around the support it has located. Finally, through a brilliant bit of botanical engineering, some tendrils are able to coil like two springs winding in opposite directions and joined midway between the plant stem and the newly found support. This creates a strong but flexible bond.

With vine spinach (*Basella alba*), on the other hand, the growing tip of the plant moves in a slow circle until it encounters a suitable structure for climbing, and then the main stem of the plant wraps tightly around it. Some climbing plants, such as grapes, need a little help. Growers will often use twist ties to hold the grape stems to the trellis until it grasps the idea. As a rule, it is good to use thick twine, rope, or wire to help plants climb because fine string and wire can cut into the stem, cutting off the circulation of nutrients as the plant gets heavier. Peas and beans are such good natural climbers that they will sometimes intertwine with their own stems making thick tangles of their vines—and in the process reduce the amount of sunshine they can harvest. Smaller openings in the trellis helps avoid this problem. Poultry netting fits the bill nicely.

Trees and trellises are not the only way to add dimension to your leafy garden. Plants can be grown in containers, and the containers can be raised on platforms, poles, fences, decks, stairs, or on roofs. They can also be hung by ropes or chains from eaves or overhangs. The foliage of plants such as sweet potato, vine spinach, Okinawa spinach, New Zealand spinach, and wolfberry can be visually compelling as it spills over the sides of a hanging container. Plants growing in hanging baskets near windows will progressively shade more of the window as the summer gets hotter.

Dig it

One of the most basic ways to add dimension and complexity to your garden is by going down, not up. As discussed earlier, building deeper soil definitely expands the possibilities of any garden. Another measure that makes for a more interesting and ecologically complete garden is digging a small pond. It doesn't need to be a formal water pond with a pump and waterfalls, as nice as those are. Just a depression in your garden lined with plastic and filled with water will quickly become home to frogs, crayfish, and be visited by toads, turtles, butterflies, skinks, salamanders, snakes, and birds. Not only will their presence make your garden a more interesting place to spend time, most of the creatures drawn to your pond will help control any insects eating your crops.

Building more dimension and complexity into your garden creates greater yields and more resilience. It brings in more life in all of its forms. This creates a spectrum of opportunities for the willing gardener to engage in an intimate ecosystem.

11

Have Your Cake and Eat It Too

❉ ❉ ❉

Growing Edible Cover Crops

Cover crops, sometimes called *fertility* or *green manure* crops, are crops grown primarily to improve soil. They increase our capacity to produce healthy food by facilitating at least six distinct chemical and physical changes in the fertility and structure of the soil (discussed below).

Cover crops are hardly a new idea. They have been used for at least 3,000 years in China and for over 2,000 years in southern Europe. Farmers have long noticed that crop yields go up in fields that had previously grown certain plants, especially plants of the legume, or pea, family. Millions of farmers over thousands of growing seasons gradually developed systems for using plants to improve the health of their soil and to produce more bountiful harvests. However, the convenience of concentrated soluble fertilizers that became widely available after World War II led to a sharp drop-off in enthusiasm for cover crops. In recent years, interest is rebounding as a growing number of farmers consider cover crops as a cheaper and more sustainable way to maintain soil fertility. Although growing cover crops is often thought of as a farm-scale technique, it is very well suited to improving the soil in home vegetable gardens. In fact, the small-scale offers gardeners the flexibility to use cover crops more creatively than is possible on the farm scale.

All cover crops are essentially leaf crops, in that they are normally mowed and used to enrich the soil before they can flower and reproduce. Once plants begin flowering and producing seed, the amount of organic matter that they can contribute to improve the soil declines significantly. Often, it is the onset of flowering that marks the optimal time to cut down cover crops.

While growing cover crops is a time-tested strategy, the idea of growing them and then eating a small portion of them is relatively new—and potentially very important. It is a way to simultaneously address two serious problems in our current food system: declining fertility and structure of our food-producing soils, and the lack of vegetables—especially leafy green vegetables—in our modern diet. Of all foods, greens provide the best ratio of nutrients per calorie, and they are excellent sources of a variety of essential vitamins, minerals, and protective antioxidants. Despite these benefits, our average consumption of leafy vegetables is less than one ounce per day.

CHON

Carbon, hydrogen, oxygen, and nitrogen make up something like 98 percent of the human body. Those four elements also make up over 95 percent of the weight of the meat, eggs, milk, grain, fruit, nuts, and vegetables that we eat. Luckily for us, all four of these are present in inexpensive and easy-to-find air and water. Air is comprised of about 78 percent nitrogen and 21 percent oxygen, with just a touch of carbon. Even with the disturbing rise in atmospheric carbon levels, carbon dioxide makes up less than 0.04 percent of the air around us. Of course, there is a lot of air. Water is about 11 percent hydrogen and 89 percent oxygen. There is a lot of water, too. In theory, we could get almost all the food we need by breathing in air and drinking water. This would do wonders for our grocery bill.

Unfortunately, only the very few most highly enlightened beings are able to get their food this way. The rest of us require that these elements be significantly modified in form before they provide us with nourishment. Plants are proficient at using the power of sunshine to modify air and water into food for people and other animals to eat. Most cover crops specialize in converting air and water into foods for *soil organisms* to eat. A well-fed soil produces more food and better quality food.

Selecting cover crops with edible leaves does reduce the number of suitable plants to choose from. Also, harvesting some portion of the crops as leaf vegetables will slow the soil-building process slightly. However, the combined payoff of abundant nutritious vegetables plus healthier, more productive soil, make edible cover crops an agricultural bargain.

Cover crops work to improve the health of soil both chemically and structurally in at least six distinct ways.

1. All cover crops add carbon to the soil, which feeds the soil food web and increases the soil organic matter. Cover crops capture carbon from the air through photosynthesis and add carbon to the soil when they are cut down and allowed to rot. Cover crops also increase soil carbon while they are alive by exuding carbon-rich sugars and starches from their roots in order to feed beneficial soil bacteria. Some researchers estimate that as much as one-quarter of the carbohydrates formed in plant leaves are exuded into the soil surrounding the roots. A third mechanism by which cover crops can add carbon to the soil is the sloughing off of roots when the above-ground plant is partially harvested. This is done by the plant in order to keep the roots and the above-ground parts of the plant in balance.

2. Leguminous cover crops in a symbiotic relationship with rhizobia soil bacteria take nitrogen from the air where plants can't use it and put it into the soil in forms that plants can absorb.

3. Some cover crops are dynamic accumulators and concentrators of essential minerals from the subsoil. For instance, mustard is an accumulator of selenium, and buckwheat accumulates phosphorus. Deep-rooted cover crops, such as alfalfa, can pull up minerals from the lower levels of the soil and leave them near the surface where they can be used and recycled by plants with shallower roots. This is important for supplying the dozen or so essential minerals that plants can't derive from air or water.

4. All cover crops physically cover bare soil and protect it from wind and water erosion. It is a key step to rebuilding functional ecosystems that provide valuable services like purifying air and water and stabilizing weather patterns. In addition, some cover crops can cover the ground so thoroughly that they not only protect against erosion but can also

completely smother out perennial weeds. This is another valuable service cover crops can perform for the gardener or farmer.

5. The extensive networks of cover crops roots, especially from grass family plants, leave miles of fine channels throughout the topsoil. These allow earthworms and other beneficial soil life to move about more freely. The channels in the soil also allow for greater movement of the air that supplies oxygen and carbon dioxide as well as the water that carries nutrients to the plants. The roots making these channels are food for a web of soil life that continually recycles and upgrades plant nutrients.

6. Cover crops with strong taproots, such as forage radishes, turnips, or sugar beets, punch holes deep into the subsoil allowing better drainage and deeper root penetration for crops that follow. A surprising member of this group of cover crop plants is the humble cowpea. Cowpeas can send a strong taproot down over seven feet in just eight weeks of growth to reach moisture and minerals unavailable to most annual plants.

Choosing Edible Cover Crops

When we are speaking of cover crops, we are almost always referring to leaf crops. While wheat is normally grown for its mature seed, and beans are usually grown for either mature seeds or immature seed pods, both wheat and beans can be grown as cover crops as well; as cover crops, though, they are normally cut down or mowed before they begin to form seeds. Plants often used as cover crops have foliage that ranges from the fairly toxic (velvet beans) to the quite delicious (Austrian winter pea). Many cover crops have edible leaves, but a smaller number have palatable leaves. My favorite edible cover crops are Austrian winter pea, cowpeas, bell beans, alfalfa, hyacinth beans, wheat, barley, turnips, forage radishes, mustard, rape, sugar beets, and sweet potatoes. The vast majority of all cover crops, and especially of edible leaf cover crops, are members of one of three plant families; the legume family, the grass family, or the mustard family.

The Legume Family

The legume family is the third-largest plant family with over 19,400 species, including familiar beans, peas, and clovers. About 185 legume species have leaves that have been eaten by humans at various times and places. Many of these edible leaf legumes make good cover crops. Most legumes have evolved symbiotic relationships with the rhizobia family of bacteria. These bacteria use an enzyme called nitrogenase to reassemble the nitrogen in the air, along with hydrogen from water, into ammonia molecules. Atmospheric nitrogen, while in great supply, is in the form of dinitrogen, or N_2, which cannot be used by plants. Once it is converted to ammonia, the nitrogen can be utilized by plants and built into an astounding array of protein molecules.

In order to maximize the amount of atmospheric nitrogen fixed (made available) to the plants that follow, legume seeds should be coated with inoculant prior to planting. Legume inoculant is live rhizobia bacteria in very finely ground peat moss. Inoculants are specific to each species of legume, but all-purpose inoculant with a mix of rhizobias for most common garden legumes can be purchased from garden supply centers or seed catalogs. If the cover crop is fixing nitrogen, it will form white or gray nodules on the roots that have a pinkish tint when broken open. Legumes will not fix nitrogen if the soil is already rich in nitrogen from fertilizer or manure.

Nitrogen is very often the factor most limiting the growth of a wide variety of food crops, and manufacturing industrial nitrogen fertilizer is the biggest single energy expense in our food system. Because of these two realities, the ability of legumes to fix atmospheric nitrogen is enormously important.

The Most Promising Edible Leguminous Cover Crops
Alfalfa (*Medicago sativa*)

Alfalfa, or lucerne, is a perennial forage plant that was first cultivated in Mesopotamia before the beginning of written history. Alfalfa is now grown throughout the world's temperate zones and the cooler parts of the tropics. It is considered to be the world's most important fodder crop.

Alfalfa's extremely deep roots (up to 30 feet) enable it to reach otherwise inaccessible nutrients from the subsoil, and to reach water during droughts. The deep roots create channels for air and water to penetrate the subsoil, improving drainage for future crops. It usually requires replanting only once every six to eight years, which greatly reduces the energy and labor costs of land preparation, and more importantly, makes alfalfa the best of all commercial crops at preventing soil erosion.

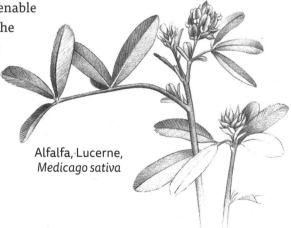

Alfalfa, Lucerne,
Medicago sativa

Alfalfa seeds are very hard and should be soaked in hot water for an hour or two before planting. Planting in ridges or rows 1.5–2 feet apart makes weeding much easier until cover is established. Leaf production is much greater if the soil has an adequate supply of phosphorus.

As just stated, alfalfa is an excellent nitrogen fixer; but it can also be harvested several times a year. Alfalfa grows well at high altitudes and in cold climates but is susceptible to viral infections in hot humid climates. In the home garden situation, it is better suited to growing in a separate patch as a fertility crop to be mowed then added to compost or used as mulch in the garden.

Alfalfa sprouts are widely eaten, and very young shoots have been eaten as potherbs in various cultures. However, the plant's potential as a direct human food has barely been touched. Unfortunately, it is too tough and stringy and sometimes too bitter to eat in the way we eat spinach or lettuce. But alfalfa can be made much more useful for direct human consumption by drying and grinding the leaves, or by converting the leaves to leaf concentrate (more on this in Chapter 12 and 13).

Cowpea (*Vigna unguiculata*)

Cowpea is a warm-weather annual legume from West Africa. The best-known type of cowpea in North America is the black-eyed pea. In addition to their dried seeds, cowpea leaves are produced as a vegetable on a commercial scale in 18 African countries and seven Asian countries. Typically, cowpeas are grown for their leaves in high rainfall areas, and for seeds in drier areas. Cowpea leaves are eaten like spinach when they are young and tender. Older leaves can be dried and used later in soups and other dishes. According to James Duke in his *Handbook of Legumes of World Economic Importance* growing cowpeas for leaves can produce, per day, nine times more calories, 15 times more protein, 90 times more calcium, and thousands of times more vitamin C and beta-carotene, than growing the same crop for seed.

Cowpeas are an excellent intercrop plant to use between rows of corn, sorghum, fruit trees, or

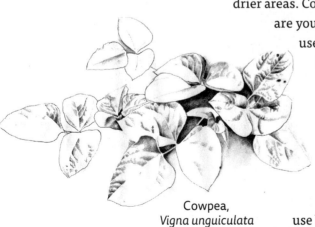

Cowpea,
Vigna unguiculata

other crops. Corn or sorghum intercropped with cowpeas will usually give about a 30 percent boost in total food yield. Both seeds and edible greens can be grown in the same garden patch by planting cowpeas in rows 16 inches apart and letting them grow till the leaves begin to touch. Then, every other row is harvested for greens without lowering seed yield. This technique allows you to capture nitrogen from the air and harvest a mild-flavored and nutritious leaf vegetable from between the rows rather than just pulling weeds. Cowpeas are a versatile fertility tool that you can plant anytime during the summer whenever a garden bed becomes open.

Cowpea seed should be soaked overnight and then inoculated with EL-type rhizobia if cowpeas haven't been grown on the land in the past three years. Actually, evidence suggests that somewhat better nitrogen fixation takes place with inoculation, even on land where cowpeas *have* been recently grown. Adding a bit of sugar to the soaked cowpeas aids inoculation by

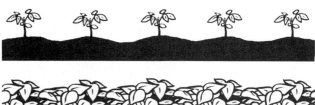

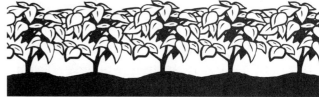

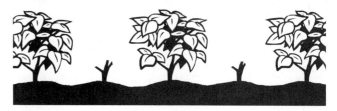

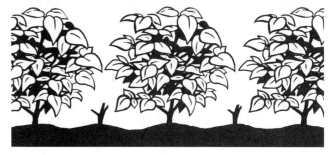

Harvest every other row when leaves begin to touch.

helping the rhizobia stick to the seeds until they sprout. "Garden mix" legume inoculants contain enough EL-type to work fine with cowpeas.

Cowpeas are sown about twice as densely for a cover crop as they are for seed production. Broadcast about ½ cup of seeds per 100-square-foot bed when grown as edible cover crops or about ¼ cup when they are grown for seeds. They can also be planted an inch deep every three inches in rows 16 inches apart. Planting in rows makes it easier to weed the bed when the plants are young.

Cowpeas are quite drought resistant as long as they get some water their first two weeks. They won't tolerate frost or being waterlogged. Plants cut at 8 inches above the ground will regrow for a second cutting, but those cut at two inches will regrow slowly if at all. In general, taking an early cutting at about three weeks after planting and then allowing the plants to begin flowering before cutting them down provides a good mix of tender young greens and a full cover crop. Forage (indeterminate) varieties of cowpeas, such as "Iron and Clay" or "Chinese Red," will produce far more foliage and are much better for cover crops than seed varieties, such as black-eyed peas.

Austrian Winter Pea (*Pisum sativa*)

Peas were one of the first plants to be cultivated by humans and are now widely grown throughout the world's temperate and sub-tropical zones. Austrian winter peas are a variety used as a cold weather cover crop to add nitrogen and organic matter to the soil. They are annual plants that grow about 24–36 inches high and have beautiful two-tone purple flowers. They don't thrive in acid or waterlogged soil, salinity, drought, or heat, but they are quite hardy in cold weather and will usually survive several freezes.

Austrian peas will produce the most biomass, soil nitrogen, and edible leaves if planted relatively early in the fall so that they can get a good measure of warmer weather and more intense sunlight. Winter peas produce nearly as well when planted in the early spring. However, spring garden planting of other crops then has to be delayed to allow the peas the time they need for generating the maximum nitrogen and biomass.

Austrian Winter Pea,
Pisum sativum

Before planting, pea seeds should be treated with pea inoculant or with an all-purpose garden inoculant. Broadcast about two ounces of seed for a 100-square-foot bed, or plant seed every five inches in rows two feet apart. There are several advantages in using close rows rather than broadcasting cover crops. Planting in rows allows you to hoe between them to reduce weed competition. It is also far easier to harvest edible leaves from rows and avoid accidentally including weeds that may not be palatable (or may even be toxic). In addition, soil improvement can be accelerated by placing organic mulch between the rows, combining the benefits of the cover crops with those of the mulch.

The tender young shoots of the pea plant have a delicious nut-like flavor and make a good salad green or potherb. Dried winter pea leaf has one of the best flavors of any dried leaf. (More information on drying leaves is coming in Chapter 12.)

A cover crop medley that provides your soil with nitrogen, organic matter, and erosion control can be established with the triple mix of Austrian winter peas, barley, and white mustard. All three of these plants have highly nutritious, edible leaves as long as they are picked when fairly young.

Other Good Edible Legume Cover Crops
Hyacinth or Lablab Bean (*Lablab purpureus*)
Lablab, or hyacinth bean, is a short-lived perennial climber native to Africa and India. It is used as a forage or cover crop as well as for its edible beans. It is a strong nitrogen fixer. Lab-labs are grown much like cowpeas but are generally more disease resistant. The purple hyacinth varieties are vigorous climbers, and their beautiful purple flowers and pods make them attractive plants for garden fences and trellises. This is a good plant for attracting hummingbirds and butterflies to a garden. Lablab thrives in a range of soil types. It is relatively drought tolerant once established, but doesn't grow well in cold weather, saline conditions, or in waterlogged soil.

Bell Bean (*Vicia faba*)
Bell bean is a small-seeded variety of the fava bean. It is a cool-weather annual usually planted in the fall or in the very early spring, though in very cold areas they are grown as a summer crop. They will usually flower within 60 days and won't regrow or reseed themselves. Young tender bell bean leaves can be eaten as a potherb or dried. They are usually too tough and strong flavored to be eaten raw.

Hyacinth Bean,
Lablab purpureus

Rice Bean (*Vigna umbellata*)

Rice beans are from India and thrive in hot, humid summers where many legume crops suffer from disease. Once established, rice beans have some resistance to drought but are sensitive to frost and waterlogging. For a cover crop, seed is normally broadcast at a rate of about two ounces per 100 square feet. The young leaves and immature pods are eaten as cooked vegetables, while the small mature beans are cooked in many rice dishes. Most varieties are vigorous climbers; the vining forms make great garden trellis plants with pretty yellow flowers.

There are many other legumes that could be used as edible leaf cover crops. These include butterfly pea (*Clitoria ternatea*), berseem clover (*Trifolium alexandrinum*), kidney bean (*Phaseolus vulgaris*), scarlet runner bean (*Phaseolus coccineus*), and fenugreek (*Trigonella foenum-graecum*).

The Grass Family

The grass family is the fourth largest of all plant families, with 10,025 known species. It is probably the most important plant family for humans, since over half of all calories consumed by humans come from the seeds of just three of these grasses: maize, wheat, and rice. Grasses grown for their edible seeds are called *cereals* or *grains*. In addition to their contribution of grains, the grass family is the second most important family of cover crops (legumes being the first). Annual grasses are commonly grown to capture carbon dioxide from the air and to build soil organic matter. Sometimes they are grown alone, but are often mixed with a legume.

A small handful of the grasses have become multi-purpose agricultural stars, providing animal feed, edible seeds, and cover crops. These include wheat, barley, oats, and rye—four of the most useful plant species on Earth. Throughout most of the US, these are often planted as cover crops in the fall after other crops are harvested. They are normally mowed in the spring and turned under or left to break down on top of the soil. Part of their great value as cover crops comes from the fact that they can be grown when most other food crops cannot.

It is often presumed that humans can eat only the dried seed of the cereal grasses, and that the leaves of the cereal plants need to be digested by ruminant animals before becoming food for us. It is true that the relatively high fiber content of grasses prevents us from using them directly as a major source of calories. However, since the 1930s, a modest amount of cereal grass leaves have been eaten by people as vegetables, revealing yet another potentially valuable use for these plants.

The nutritional profile of young cereal grasses is actually quite similar to that of most nutritious dark green leafy vegetables, all of which are rich in chlorophyll, high in fiber, and best eaten before the plant begins to flower. While fiber is indigestible by humans, the relatively high fiber content of these green leafy foods is actually beneficial for people eating a modern industrial diet. North Americans typically consume less than half the recommended plant fiber. For people on these diets, doubling the average intake of dietary fiber would lower rates of digestive disorders, obesity, some cancers, diabetes, and heart disease.

Cereal grasses, especially wheat and barley, have been marketed almost entirely through health food outlets, mostly as supplements rather than as foods. Exaggerated claims about their healing powers—and even more exaggerated prices—have limited their appeal to the small but growing segment of the populace that is extremely concerned with nutrition.

While cereal grasses are expensive to buy, gardeners can cheaply and easily incorporate them into their food systems. They are very productive and easily grown crops that can provide substantial amounts of beta-carotene, vitamin K, folic acid, calcium, iron, protein, fiber, vitamin C, and many of the B vitamins. When grown in the home garden, they provide all of these at a very low cost. Seed for wheat and barley greens is very cheap compared to most other dark green leafy vegetables. These cereals are less labor intensive because they have relatively few problems with insect pests, and they can be grown when the garden is not needed for other crops.

Growing the young cereal grasses for leaf vegetables combined with growing them as soil-improving cover crops is a winning combination. Most of the research, development, and marketing has been concerned with wheat and barley grasses. They are very similar crops in terms of how they grow and how they can be eaten.

Wheat (*Triticum aestivum, Triticum durum*)
Barley (*Hordeum vulgare*)

Wheat and barley originated in western Asia. Their domestication in the valleys of the Tigris and Euphrates Rivers roughly 10,000–12,000 years ago is considered by many to mark the beginning of agriculture and civilization. The cultivation of these two cereals has spread from that fertile crescent to most of the world's temperate and sub-tropical regions. Wheat now ranks just behind maize and just ahead of rice among the world's most produced food crops.

Wheat and barley are impressive multi-use plants. Their fibrous mats of roots loosen up tough soils and feed earthworms and soil bacteria, while their abundant production of biomass fixes carbon from the air as beneficial organic matter for the soil. They produce huge yields of nutritious greens with almost no waste. Cereal grasses make excellent fodder for animals either fresh or dried as hay. If some of the crop is allowed to mature, it will yield nutritious whole grains. And when the grain is separated from the stalks, the leftover straw makes excellent mulch or animal bedding. There is also a burgeoning interest in building houses with straw bales (in spite of *The Three Little Pigs'* warning).

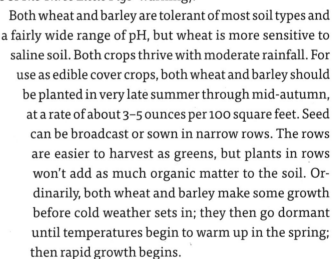

Barley and Wheat,
Hordeum vulgare and
Triticum aestivum,
Triticum durum

Both wheat and barley are tolerant of most soil types and a fairly wide range of pH, but wheat is more sensitive to saline soil. Both crops thrive with moderate rainfall. For use as edible cover crops, both wheat and barley should be planted in very late summer through mid-autumn, at a rate of about 3–5 ounces per 100 square feet. Seed can be broadcast or sown in narrow rows. The rows are easier to harvest as greens, but plants in rows won't add as much organic matter to the soil. Ordinarily, both wheat and barley make some growth before cold weather sets in; they then go dormant until temperatures begin to warm up in the spring; then rapid growth begins.

For a cover crop or for leafy vegetables, wheat or barley should be harvested just before the reproductive cycle—*the jointing process*—begins. Beds can be mowed with a heavy-duty lawn mower, a string weed cutter, or a scythe. Like most cover crops, the cut wheat plants can be incorporated into the top few inches of the soil with a tiller or hoe, hauled off to use as mulch or compost elsewhere, or simply allowed to rot in place. The rot-in-place alternative is becoming popular because it gives the best soil protection and takes the least work. Also, when cover crops are tilled or plowed under they are less accessible to the aerobic bacteria that are concentrated in the very top layer of the soil and are best suited for rapidly breaking down crop residues. The rot-in-place option works better when robust transplants (tomatoes, peppers, or sweet potatoes, for example) or large-seeded crops are planted in the residue, rather than small-seeded crops.

The ability of a cover crop to improve the soil will be somewhat diminished when a portion of the crop is used directly as food rather than left in the field. However, the loss of soil building can be minimal if only 20–30 percent of the above-ground crop is used as food. In any case, much of the benefit of cereal cover crops comes from the roots, which improve soil structure.

The yields of cover crops can vary considerably depending on soil and weather conditions, timing, and density of planting. A typical cover crop of wheat might produce 4,000 pounds of wheat grass per acre. This comes out to about nine pounds for a 100-square-foot bed. If 20 percent is removed as leaf and the remaining 80 percent allowed to enrich the soil, nearly two pounds of dried wheat grass may be reaped from an average-sized garden bed. When you consider that dried wheat grass and barley grass is often sold for $20 a pound (or more) by health food retailers, this looks like an economical proposition. Fresh or cooked wheat and barley grass tends to be stringy, but dried and powdered they are a mild-flavored and super-nutritious addition to many dishes (drying and powdering are discussed in Chapter 12).

The Mustard Family

There are about 3,700 species in the mustard family, most of them native to the Mediterranean region. They are now widely grown throughout the temperate zones and the cooler parts of the tropics. Many members of this Brassica family, sometimes referred to as the mustard or cabbage family, are valuable and familiar foods. This clan includes broccoli, cauliflower, Brussels sprouts, kale, kohlrabi, mustard, turnips, radishes, rape (Canola), watercress, and the familiar head cabbage. They are all rich in beta-carotene, vitamin C, potassium, calcium, and boron (an important mineral for strong bones). They contain sulphoraphane and indoles, effective cancer-fighting antioxidants, as well as a substance that helps protect our stomach lining from acid and eases the pain of ulcers.

Many varieties of turnip, mustard, radish, and rape have been used as cover crops. None of these fix nitrogen, as legumes do, but all four have deep roots that help break up compacted soil, and all four add a significant amount of organic matter to the soil. A further advantage of mustard family cover crops is that they can reduce pest problems for the crops that follow them. The same sulfur compounds that provide the snappy flavor and the nutritional protection against cancer also inhibit the growth of many crop diseases and nematodes. Turnips, mustards, radishes, and rape can be used alone as cover crops or they can be combined with legumes and/or grasses for a more complete green manure.

Common mustard family cover crops:
- Turnips *Brassica rapa* var. *rapa*
- Rape or Canola *Brassica napus*
- White mustard *Brassica hirta*
- Field mustard *Brassica campestris*
- Brown mustard *Brassica juncea*
- Black mustard *Brassica nigra*
- Fodder radish *Raphanus sativus*

All of the mustard family cover crops are cool-weather plants that can be sown in early spring or in late summer for a fall crop. All germinate quickly. Seed for turnip and mustard can be broadcast at about an ounce per 100 square feet, or planted in rows 18 inches apart and thinned to every three inches. Fodder radish requires about twice as much seed, but rape requires only about one-third as much. Dragging the back end of a rake lightly over the seed covers it and assures good soil contact.

Turnips and fodder radishes have especially strong and deep tap roots, sometimes drilling 6–9 feet into the soil. Canola is a type of rape seed that has been bred to produce a healthier cooking oil. Most rape is now genetically modified, though the extra price of the seed makes it of less value for use as a cover crop. Essex Dwarf is a cheap, non-GMO variety of rape that makes an excellent cover crop with tasty greens.

Some mustard varieties can produce up to 30 pounds of biomass per 100-square-foot bed in just five weeks. A cover crop of mustard is considered to be especially beneficial when turned in before a crop of potatoes because it reduces many of the diseases affecting potatoes.

Thinnings from any of these mustard family cover crops make good greens. Turnip greens are a traditional dish in the southeastern US. The tiny hairs (technically, "trichomes") on the leaves disappear with cooking. Newer, tender leaves can still be harvested from the center as the plants begin to mature, but once flowering begins, all the leaves become quite tough and bitter. Only the very youngest leaves are eaten raw. Of course, harvesting leaves will somewhat reduce the amount of biomass returned to the soil. Optimal proportions of leaf harvest, root harvest, green manure, and even seed harvest will need to be determined based on the specifics of each crop and each garden situation.

How to Grow Edible Cover Crops

For most of North America, the best time to grow cover crops is often over the winter when the garden is idle. Usually two or three weeks before the first expected frost is a good time to plant so that the cover crop has time to establish some roots before hard freezes come.

A good mix of edible winter cover crops is wheat, Austrian winter peas, and turnips. They can be planted in adjacent strips but the seed can also just be mixed and broadcast together. All three have edible high-nutrition leaves, and research is showing that the combination of the three is much better at soil building than each of them separately.

The practice of mixing members of the three basic cover crop families— legume, grass, and mustard—goes back to an old German agricultural system called *Landsberger Gemenge*. The idea was that three or sometimes even four different crops together would produce a mixture that is very nutritious and well-balanced for feeding cattle and sheep, as well as the soil. By choosing edible varieties, you are able to produce food for livestock, the soil, and the dinner table—a veritable land salad.

Backyard gardeners may think they don't have enough space to grow cover crops, edible or otherwise. On very small lots this may be true, but often there is a pre-existing cover crop growing in the form of a lawn. With a few adjustments, lawns can be managed to support the fertility of kitchen gardens. It is important to incorporate legumes such as clovers with the grasses so that the lawn/cover crop can become self-sustaining in terms of nitrogen. Such a lawn/cover crop would be able to produce plenty of organic matter indefinitely as long as soil minerals are periodically replaced.

In practice, it is difficult to grow a lawn as an *edible* cover because lawns are normally exposed to much more foot traffic than one would expect in a garden bed. It is, however, very possible to grow a combination lawn/cover crop twice the size of your vegetable garden that will maintain the fertility of that garden. When you mow the grass/cover crop lawn, add the clippings to the vegetable garden as mulch or use them to make compost for the garden.

Pet Peeves

It is important to be aware of dog (especially puppy) and cat feces on lawns that might contaminate clippings with the eggs of parasitic roundworms. These can lie dormant for a long time and don't break down easily, even in compost piles. Also, backyard gardeners may have heard horror stories of vegetable crops ruined by the residues of herbicides from lawn clippings used as mulch or in compost.

The problem is with a particular class of long-lasting, resistant herbicides that include clopyralid. Most home lawns won't have clopyralid because it has not been registered for use on residential lawns in the US since 2002. But golf courses and other institutions still commonly use these herbicides, and grass clippings from them is not worth using unless you know for sure that the herbicides haven't been used. These herbicides are very slow to degrade and can show up in hay from treated fields or even in manure from animals that have eaten hay from treated fields. Until these troubling poisons are completely outlawed, it pays to exercise caution when bringing grass clippings, hay, or manure into your garden.

Problems can be avoided by following the principle promoted by many ecological agriculture advocates of making your garden or farm as self-sustaining as possible. Some supporters of this approach says that the importation of nutrients just robs organic matter and minerals from some other place; all you are doing is simply relocating the soil deficit. The logic is solid, but in our modern world there is significant movement of organic matter that won't be alleviated by self-contained farms. Raked up and bagged autumn leaves, grass clippings, and brush cleared from roadsides and utility lines are treated as waste—and sometimes hauled long distances—to be buried in landfills. Clearly, this is a shortsighted plan, so shouldn't gardeners take advantage of these resources to build their garden soil, rather than adhere to a strict agricultural ideology?

Learning how to grow and use edible cover crops seems like a reasonable strategy to minimize problems with imported fertility while simultaneously improving the diet and health of the gardener's family by putting more green leafy vegetables on the dinner table.

Edible Cover Crop Math

Average home vegetable garden is 600 square feet, or 24 × 25 feet, or 1/70 acre.

Let's assume a gardener wants to maximize his or her leaf harvests. In the autumn, after most of the summer vegetables were done growing, most of the garden would be planted in Austrian winter peas, barley, and mixed members of the Brassica family (kale, rape, mustard, turnips, radish, etc.). Let's say 200 square feet each in winter peas and barley, and 100 square feet of brassica plants. These would be mowed down in the early spring, and 100 square feet of bell bean cover crop could be planted before space was needed for warm season crops like sweet potatoes and tomatoes. In the remaining 200 square feet of garden, potatoes, cabbage, beets, carrots and other spring and early summer crops would be planted. After they were harvested, they would be replaced with a cover crop of cowpeas. Because cowpeas grow fast in summer heat, 200 square feet of them could be grown by simply broadcasting their seed wherever a space opened up. When the cowpeas came out, it would be nearly time for winter cover crops to go in.

By growing cover crops year round this gardener would produce about 600 pounds of above-ground cover crop each year. Assuming half that total was stem, about 300 pounds of edible leaf crop would be available. If the gardener took 100 pounds (one-third) of the leaf as food, 200 pounds of leaf could still be returned to the soil as mulch or compost. In addition, the 300 pounds of stems and all of the roots would also be returned to soil to help build soil organic matter.

The 100 pounds of fresh greens is about five times our current average annual consumption of greens, so it could potentially play a large role in improving our diet. The extra servings of greens could move people much closer to the World Health Organization's recommendation to eat at least 600 grams (about one and a third pounds) of fruits and vegetables daily in order to minimize the risk of cancers, heart disease, and diabetes. This nutritional bonus could be added to the family's pantry essentially without cost and without the need to add any additional growing space and *at the same time* it would significantly improve the garden's productive capacity.

12

What Lasts Is Not Least

❈ ❈ ❈

Preserving the Leaf Harvest

In parts of Central America, May through September are "los meses flacos," the skinny months. In Kenya, May and June are sometimes referred to as "Wanjala" or hunger season. And in the Rangpur region of Bangladesh, September to November is known as "mora Kartik," the months of death and disaster. Most of the serious hunger in the world is seasonal and fairly predictable.

The reasons for this are rooted in agricultural and biological economics. The demand for food is very inelastic, nearly constant. Everybody wants to eat every single day. The supply of food is quite variable; usually the greatest after the harvest and the smallest just before the next harvest. Since demand is nearly constant, the price of food tends to be lowest after the harvest and highest before the next harvest. That is when poor people can't afford enough food and the cycle of hunger begins to repeat itself.

Food is created by photosynthesis. Almost everywhere, the bulk of food is produced during the three months with the best combination of warmth and soil moisture for efficient photosynthesis. For everyone to eat every day requires us to find ways to capture the sunlight from those warm, moist days as food and move it around in space and time in order to reach everyone's dinner plate. This is an undertaking central to the success of the human species.

The industrial food system does two important things to prevent recurrent seasonal hunger. First of all, it preserves food from the harvest so that it can be eaten all year. Secondly, it moves food from areas of high supply and low demand, typically rural agricultural regions, to areas of low supply and high demand. Increasingly, these are urban areas where little food is grown but much is eaten.

Within industrialized societies, most of us are fairly well protected from seasonal hardships. Buildings, and even cars, are heated during cold weather and cooled during hot spells. Water is piped inside whether it rains outside or not. In a drought, we may be discouraged from washing cars or watering lawns, but there is usually plenty of water for bathing and washing dishes and clothes. We are especially well insulated from seasonal food shortages. Fresh corn on the cob, tomatoes, and watermelon are cheaper and better quality in season, but overall the price and availability of food doesn't change much over the course of a year. As long as the global food economy is functioning and you have the money to participate, the seasons are largely irrelevant.

Of course, the situation looks very different when thinking about *local* food systems. Farmers markets may be flooded with relatively inexpensive sweet corn and tomatoes for six weeks in late summer. They may be available at a premium price for several weeks before and after the peak. Then they are gone. This does not bring on months of "death and disaster" as it might in developing countries because of paid off-farm work and functional, if frayed, social safety nets. However, this seasonality of farm income and of fresh food availability is a serious constraint to the growth of local food economies.

Many small-scale farmers are earning extra income by stretching their growing seasons with hoop houses or high tunnels. These are inexpensive unheated greenhouses that provide enough protection from the cold to significantly lengthen the season for many crops. This enables farmers to increase their income and to increase the availability of fresh produce in their communities. Some farmers are also trying to spread their peak harvest periods over the whole year by preserving produce. Converting excess produce into jams, pickles, sauces, and other foods can generate a small but important income flow. Increasing the shelf life of locally grown produce also reduces the amount of food that communities need to bring in from afar.

No one imagines that hot sauce, jam, and chutney will feed a town, but preserving extra food produced during peak growing seasons rather than letting it go to waste—as is now often the case—is just sound economics.

The effort to diversify agricultural income and increase the percentage of locally grown food we eat is a significant one. It is a fundamental reality in Nicaragua, Kenya, and Bangladesh, but it is also important in Ohio, Ontario, and everywhere people aspire to build vigorous, self-reliant communities.

As with pickles and jellies, leafy green vegetables alone won't feed a town. However, unlike condiments, greens could become the primary dietary source of many essential nutrients. A plentiful year-round supply of nutritious locally produced leaf vegetables would be a big step toward food self-sufficiency for any community. Chapter 9 of this book discussed how to keep fresh greens on your table by extending their normal growing season. This chapter explains how to preserve some of the fresh greens that you grow in order to have them available all year round.

Why Do You Have To Preserve Food?

Why can't you just set it aside and come back three months later and eat it? Two different things cause food to spoil or rot: microbes eating the food and multiplying, and enzymes within the food causing various components of the food to break down into less delicious compounds. The largely microscopic spoilage organisms are the bigger problem. They are endemic, that is, they are essentially everywhere. In the nearly ideal conditions provided by warm moist food, the population of the bacteria, molds, and fungi that are competing with us for that food can multiply with geometric intensity. Their presence in large numbers changes the flavor, texture, and nutritional value of foods. Some of these microbes, such as salmonella and listeria, can cause food poisoning.

Enzymes are not alive; they are proteins that act as catalysts accelerating chemical reactions or allowing reactions to take place with lower energy inputs. After a plant is harvested, many enzymes in the food speed its rate of spoilage. For example, an enzyme called polyphenol oxidase causes sliced apples and potatoes to turn brown. Lipoxidases are enzymes that speed up the oxidization of lipids, or oils, in green vegetables, which imparts an unpleasant fishy flavor.

Over thousands of years, we have developed several strategies for minimizing microbial growth on our food. The simplest and likely earliest food preservation technique was sun-drying. Bacteria need water to grow. Drying food below 12 percent moisture slows bacterial growth to a crawl. As we moved away from the sunny tropics, we added smoke-drying to our food preservation toolkit. Gradually, we learned to keep food by packing it in salt and sugars. Both salt and sugar in sufficient concentration will draw enough moisture through the cell walls of spoilage microbes to kill them or at least slow their growth. Salt pork, pickles, jams, and jellies are preserved in this way.

Canning preserves food by first heating it to the point of killing all the bacteria present then sealing it in an airtight glass or metal container to exclude new bacteria. Some bacteria—including the one that causes deadly botulism—must be heated well above the boiling point of water. This is usually accomplished by heating water under pressure in a specialized canner.

Some foods can be preserved by lowering the pH with vinegar or with lactic acid-forming bacteria. Yogurt, sauerkraut, and kimchi are made in this way. Most bacteria can't reproduce in environments that are very acidic. Refrigeration and freezing preserve food by slowing all of the biological processes of the spoilage organisms. Fortunately, drying, canning, and freezing not only stop microbial growth but also neutralize or deactivate most of the enzymes responsible for food spoilage.

When it comes to leaf vegetables, some of the different food preservation techniques fare far better than others. Below is my general assessment:

- Sugar, salt, and smoke reduce the nutritional value of the leaves too much and add anti-nutritional factors. *Not recommended.*
- Canning damages the nutritional value, flavor, and texture of the leaves. *Not recommended.*
- Fermentation alters the flavors and nutritional value of the leaves. Some vitamin A and vitamin C is lost during fermentation process, but B vitamins and protein quality are usually improved. The length of time fermented leaf vegetables remain good without refrigeration is quite variable, and the process often adds excess salt. *Recommended with caution on excessive salt.*
- Freezing preserves the original quality and nutritional value of the leaves best of all the commonly used techniques. It's long-term preservation, but not everyone has a freezer with adequate space, and it is an energy-intensive way to store food. *Recommended for people with adequate freezer space, though not very energy efficient.*
- Drying alters the texture and flavor of leaves. Some vitamin C and

vitamin A in the leaves is lost. Drying is simple and can be done with a low-cost homemade solar leaf dryer. Dried leaves will keep for up to a year with no energy costs. Dried leaves can be easily ground and used in a large variety of dishes. *Recommended.*

Fermenting Leaf Vegetables

Fermenting leaves generally uses cultures of lactobacilli to make the leaves too acidic for spoilage bacteria to reproduce. A recipe for the famous Korean fermented leaf dish, kimchi is given in the recipe section. Below are basic instructions for making sauerkraut (fermented cabbage).

1. Shred 5 pounds of cabbage into thin strips.
2. Mix cabbage thoroughly with 3 tablespoons of kosher or sea salt. Let sit for 5 minutes.
3. Pack cabbage/salt mixture tightly into 3 or 4 wide-mouth quart jars.
4. Pour any extra brine over the cabbage.
5. Put smaller jars (jelly jars) weighted with rocks inside the canning jars to hold the cabbage below the level of the brine.
6. Cover the jar with a cloth secured by a rubber band to allow air in but keep dust out.
7. Press the smaller jars into the cabbage twice a day and make sure the cabbage is covered with brine.
8. Allow it to ferment at room temperature. After 3 days, begin tasting it every day until it tastes right to you.
9. Remove the smaller, rock-filled jar, then screw the lid on the larger jar and refrigerate. It should keep at least two months in a refrigerator. Throw out if it turns brown.

Freezing Leaf Vegetables

Directions for freezing greens are widely available through agricultural extension offices or through the National Center for Home Food Preservation at nchfp.uga.edu. The six steps below summarize the preferred technique.

1. Wash leaves and remove stems.
2. Cut into bite-sized pieces.
3. Blanch 2 minutes (3 minutes for heavy greens like kale or wolfberry). Use a gallon of water for each 2 cups of cut greens.
4. Put greens in ice water for 2 minutes.

5. Drain thoroughly and pack tightly in freezer bags or containers.
6. Frozen greens will keep well for 1–1½ years at 0°F.

Solar Drying Leaf Vegetables

Compared to meat or fish or fruit, green leaves are simple to dry. Because leaves usually form as thin sheets for better sunshine collection, no part of the leaf is far from the surface, and the surface is where water evaporates. Three things speed leaf drying, and they are familiar to anyone who has dried clothes on a clothes line.

1. *Temperature:* Clothes dry faster on a warm day.
   The ideal temperature for drying leaves is about 130°F (55°C).
2. *Air Flow:* Clothes dry faster on a breezy, warm day.
   As air around the dryer is heated, it becomes less dense and rises. This draws more air past the leaves, replacing the humid air surrounding the leaves with drier air. If temperature exceeds 130°F, increase airflow both to speed drying and to prevent overheating.
3. *Surface Area:* Clothes dry faster if you spread them out, increasing their surface area.
   Water evaporates from the surface of leaves. As the surface becomes dry, moisture from deeper in the leaves migrates to the surface where it too can evaporate. Chopping the leaves increases their surface area and so speeds drying time. Spreading the leaves more thinly on the drying tray is the simplest way to increase surface area.

Quality Control

Leaf vegetables have been dried for thousands of years and are still being dried using traditional methods in some parts of the world. Unfortunately, the quality of traditionally dried leaves is usually poor. There are two major problems. First, the valuable beta-carotene in the leaves is almost completely destroyed when leaves are dried in full sunlight. Indirect sunlight—even the amount found indoors or in shade—has enough UV radiation to greatly reduce the vitamin A activity of the leaves. Secondly, dried leaf produced with traditional methods is often contaminated with excessive bacteria, yeast, or mold growth. Drying the leaves in the shade lessens the first problem, but the longer drying time gives the microbes and the enzymes more time to do damage before leaves are fully dry.

Heat for Food Dryers

Electric Heat: There are many small electric food dehydrators, or dryers, on the market, and plans for building your own can be easily found on the Internet. They usually have an electrical resistance heating element, and a fan to increase airflow. The best ones, like Excalibur, have thermostats to control the temperature and horizontal (rather than vertical) airflow. They cost about $200 and can dry two pounds of fresh leaves in five or six hours. Electric dehydrators are capable of drying leaves at night and in any sort of weather. The big advantages of electric dehydrators are good temperature control and convenience. The downsides are initial costs and ongoing operating costs. Cheap electric food dryers with the heater at the bottom are much less effective.

Wood Heat: It is difficult to control the drying temperature and to keep wood smoke from affecting the flavor and damaging the quality of the leaves being dried. As well, wood is often burned at too low a temperature, resulting in local air pollution.

Solar Heat: There are dozens of designs for solar-powered food dryers in all sizes and levels of complexity. The main benefit of solar dehydrators is that they use only the free non-polluting energy of sunshine. Their biggest drawback is that they don't work when the sun isn't shining. Most solar dehydrators use glass or plastic to trap heat from the sun and rely on the heated air rising to create airflow.

Much higher-quality dried leaf vegetables can be made by applying three principles: dry leaves out of sunlight; dry leaves in one day; and blanch leaves before drying.

Don't dry leaves in sunlight! When leaves are dried in sunlight, the dark green color quickly fades to a paler grayish green. This is caused mainly by high-energy ultraviolet rays in the sunlight breaking apart molecules of the chlorophyll and carotenoid pigments that give the leaves their characteristic color. Not only is the color of the faded leaves less appealing, but most of their vitamin A value is destroyed. Use sunshine as a *source* of heat for the dryer, but don't dry leaves in direct sunlight.

Dry leaves in a single day. Adjust the amount of leaves to be dried to the temperature and humidity, so that single-day drying can be accomplished. Leaves left out on dryers overnight tend to reabsorb moisture as the temperature drops. This makes them more prone to mold.

Heat leaves before drying. Heating leaves for three minutes in steam kills pathogens and improves the flavor and nutritional quality of dried leaves. This is especially important for dried leaves that will be stored for more than 1 month. Leaves can also be heated for 3–5 minutes in a microwave oven, depending on the wattage of the microwave.

How to Build a Simple and Inexpensive Solar Dryer for Leaves

When sunshine is plentiful and the air is warm, a very simple inexpensive solar dryer design will work fine for drying leaves (but not for drying fruit, meat, or fish). Because most leaves are thin sheets, they are one of the easiest foods to dry. This design described below enlarges the solar collection area to match the area of the drying tray. It has a single drying tray that allows air to pass freely both under and over the drying leaves. By enlarging the ratio of collector area to dryer area and removing obstacles to free air flow, this dryer will normally dry leaves completely in one day.

The dryer usually costs less than $20 and can be built in an hour with common hand tools. The best material for the top of the dryer is usually greenhouse-grade, 6-mil polyethylene sheeting. This lets sunlight energy in, but blocks carotene-damaging UV radiation. It is inexpensive, tough, and easy to work with. This type of greenhouse plastic is intended to last four years, though keeping the dryer out of sunlight when not in use will extend the life of the polyethylene. You can get greenhouse plastic at some farm supply stores or through greenhouse supply stores on the Internet. Greenhouse owners often have a bit left over that they may sell or give to you. It is important that you not use "regular" polyethylene sheeting because it does not block out the UV and will quickly photo-degrade and crumble.

1. Start by making two identical wooden frames. They can be any size that is convenient between 24" × 30" and 40" × 40". Larger sizes are harder to handle on a windy day, but they can dry more leaves. It is relatively cheap and easy to work with 2" × 2" framing lumber.

2. To make the base, or bottom, of your dryer, stretch ¼" hardware cloth or strong plastic pet screen tight over one of the frames and staple all around the edges. Then nail diagonal braces over the screen.

3. Reinforce the corners of the other frame (the cover, or top) to make sure frame stays square. This can be done with angle braces.

4. Stretch 6-mil greenhouse polyethylene tight and staple it to the top frame. Double the plastic where you staple for extra strength.

5. Staple a 4" strip of dark-colored, open weave cloth to each side of the dryer cover. This lets you raise the cover a bit on very hot days for greater air flow, but keeps insects and dust out.

6. Dryer is ready to use!

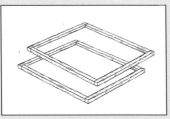

Start by making two identical wooden frames.

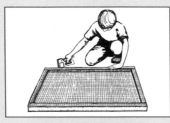

Staple or nail coarse screen to base.

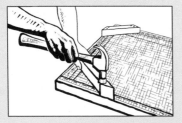

Nail diagonal braces over the coarse screen on the base.

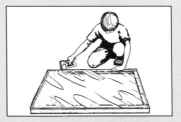

Staple or nail greenhouse plastic onto the top.

Variations on the Simple Solar Leaf Dryer

Black Sheet Metal Cover: Old sheet metal roofing sanded and then painted a flat black can be substituted for the greenhouse sheeting. Sunshine will heat the black metal and some of that heat will pass through to warm the leaves in the dryer tray. The metal will completely block UV radiation. These dryers will perform nearly as well as those covered in greenhouse plastic on clear hot days, but don't do as well on cloudy days.

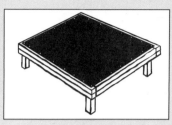

Use old metal roofing where greenhouse plastic is not available. It should be painted with non-reflective black paint.

Reflectors: Placing a shiny reflector behind your dryer will increase heat and speed drying. Reflectors are especially useful on partially cloudy days and in cooler temperatures. New galvanized sheet metal or old metal roofing painted with chrome paint from an auto

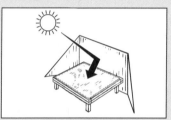

Shiny metal can reflect extra sunshine onto the dryer.

parts store works well. A piece of this reflective roofing roughly the same size as the dryer can be held behind the dryer by two fins of the same sheet metal cut at 45° angles (see drawing). A bit of testing will help determine the optimal position for a reflector in your location. The reflector needs to be stabilized so it doesn't fly off in the wind. A reflector can also make up for the slight loss of performance in using a black metal top rather than treated polyethylene.

Ant Traps: Where ants are a major problem, you can protect your drying leaves by raising the dryer on short legs and putting the legs in food cans or plastic cups filled with water. Scraps of plastic plumbing pipe make good legs because they don't rot in the water.

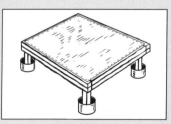

Cups of water keep ants from entering the leaf dryer.

How to Use a Simple Solar Leaf Dryer

1. If the solar dryer will be on the ground, put a sheet of plastic on the ground below the dryer to block moisture rising from the soil. Set up the solar dryer where it will have full sunshine all day and is away from animals and playing children. Raise the base of the dryer off the ground by placing it on bricks or blocks to make sure that air can move below the dryer. Raise the side of the dryer that faces away from the noon sun (north, in the Northern Hemisphere) a bit higher for a more direct solar angle and to drain unexpected rain. Do not raise it so much that the leaves will slide to the low slide as they dry. If the outdoor temperature is over 90°F, the dryer may get too hot. In this case, separate the dryer's base and cover with small wooden blocks to create more air flow and reduce the temperature.

2. Harvest and wash leaves in clean water. Remove large stems, roots, rocks, weeds, etc. The stems of leaves have little nutritional value. Removing them will speed drying and make a more nutritionally dense leaf powder.

3. Cut leaves into pieces no longer than your thumb. This increases surface area and makes for faster, more even leaf drying.

4. Blanch leaves in steam or in a microwave oven for 3 minutes. This step is especially important if the dried leaf powder will be stored for several months.

5. Spread leaves evenly in dryer in the morning so they can fully dry in one day. Between 2–3 pounds of fresh cut leaves per square yard (36" on a side) of dryer is usually about the maximum. Too thick a layer of leaves will keep the dryer too cool, and some leaves could spoil before they dry.

6. Check on the leaves in mid-afternoon if possible. Reposition the leaves so they will dry evenly.

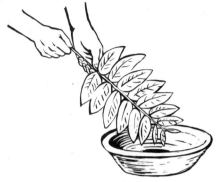

Strip leaves from stem.

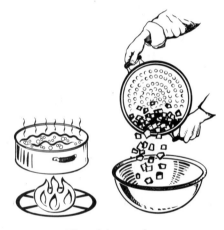

Blanch leaves for
three minutes in steam.

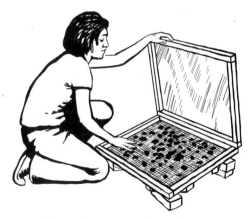

Spread leaves evenly on dryer.

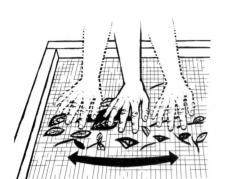

Rub the dried leaves through a coarse screen to remove as much of the remaining stems as possible.

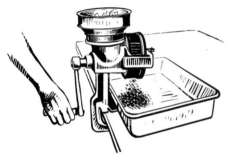

Grind dried leaves into fine powder with manual grain grinder.

7. When leaves are dry enough to be uniformly brittle, carefully remove them from the dryer and sift them by rubbing them through a metal screen to remove additional fibrous stems and leaf mid-ribs that weren't stripped off before drying. One-quarter inch hardware cloth or mesh works well.

8. Grind the sifted leaves to a fine powder. You can easily do this in a hand-cranked corn mill, an electric grain grinder, a coffee mill, a household blender, or a traditional stone grinder. Make sure leaves are very dry or they will clog the grinders. With some grinders, you will need to grind the leaves more than once, using progressively finer settings. If the leaves are uncomfortably hot to touch from grinding, slow the grinding down a bit to prevent breakdown of nutrients and flavor.

    Grinding is an important step. Finely ground dried leaves have more surface area to come into contact with digestive enzymes, and powdered leaves' nutrients are better absorbed than with coarsely ground leaves.

9. Make sure dried leaves are crisp before storing. It is important to lower the moisture content of the leaves quickly over the first 8 hours to minimize spoilage. Crisp leaves will generally contain too little moisture (less than 12 percent) to support the growth of molds and bacteria. Technically inclined gardeners can determine the moisture content by drying a sample thoroughly in a warm oven and comparing the fresh weight to the dried weight. But crispness is generally an adequate measure of proper moisture content.

Aflatoxins are naturally occurring toxins that are produced by many species of aspergillus fungi. Aflatoxins are toxic to the liver and among the most carcinogenic substances known. Grains, peanuts, and other oilseeds that have not been adequately dried are among the foods most frequently contaminated with aflatoxin.

Higher Performance Solar Food Dryer

In areas that are cool or cloudy much of the year, a somewhat more complex and expensive solar dryer will work better than the simple leaf dryer. This dryer uses a solar collector area three times larger than the area of the drying tray to increase the heat flowing to the leaves. It also has a more efficient mechanism for capturing solar heat and channeling it both over and under the drying leaves. This dryer has a thermometer to monitor the temperature near the drying tray and adjustable vents at the top and bottom to better control air flow and heat. It is more difficult to build and more difficult to move around than the simple two-piece dryer, but it can sustain higher temperatures. This means it is also useful for drying fruits, which isn't the case with the simpler, smaller dryer.

Step-by-step instructions for building and using this solar leaf dryer can be found and downloaded from the Leaf for Life website: leafforlife.org/PDFS/english/5-a-day_sun-dried_way.pdf.

How to Use Dried Leaves

1. The nutritional value of many recipes can be enhanced by replacing some of the ingredients with dried leaf powder. Usually about 20 percent of the flour in most recipes can be replaced with leaf powder without an unacceptable effect on flavor or texture. Use leaf powder from mild-flavored greens in sweet dishes or foods being made for children, and stronger-flavored greens when chili, garlic, curry, ginger, and other spices will mask the stronger flavors.

2. Cookies in the shape of dinosaurs, frogs, and Christmas trees, which would normally be green, are great ways to introduce children to leaf-powder foods. Green birthday cakes have also been a big hit. Green pasta is another readily accepted food. A child will often gladly eat two ounces of enriched pasta, although he might refuse to eat greens. If the pasta is 20 percent leaf powder, a serving will have roughly the equivalent of a whole serving of fresh greens. Children seem to especially enjoy eating pasta that they have helped to make. Recipes for dinosaur cookies, birthday cakes, and instruction for making green pasta are in the recipe section of this book (Chapter 14).

3. Keep leaf powder in a tightly sealed container, away from light and in a cool place. Use within one year.

Dry Weight

There is a great deal of confusion, some of it intentional, around the issue of dry versus wet weight. For example, an impressive graphic that has been copied by hundreds of groups compares the nutrients in moringa favorably to those in oranges, carrots, milk, bananas, and yogurt. The problem is that the comparisons are between dried moringa leaf and foods that haven't been dried. Measuring the calcium in dried moringa leaf against that in dried milk powder, or the calcium in fresh moringa versus that in fresh milk, would make for more realistic, if less impressive, comparisons. (The nutritional value of moringa is excellent; no need to tilt the board in its favor.)

It is worth noting that many of the differences in the nutritional values of fresh green leaves are mainly differences in the amount of water in them. Edible fresh leaf crops average about 89 percent moisture. Leaves that have less-than-average water, such as moringa, appear especially nutritious. Leaves that contain more than an average amount of moisture, such as vine spinach, appear to be less nutritious. However, if you remove the water, which has no nutritive value, they are very similar. So, the composition of dried leaf powder from different plants is much more similar than the composition of their fresh leaves.

It might surprise most people to know that on a dry-weight basis, several types of green leaves have higher protein content than cheddar cheese or raw hamburger, and nearly as high as eggs. For example, thoroughly dried moringa leaf is about 45 percent protein, while dried cheddar cheese is about 40 percent protein and dried whole milk is about 27 percent protein.

Leaf Powders

Dried leaf powders could potentially add a valuable new product to local food economies. In the same way that raisins are not grapes, dried leaf is a different product than fresh leaf. Once dried, the desperate urgency of moving the leaf crop from the field to the table could give way to a more relaxed pace that can extend through the entire year.

Another advantage of drying leaf crops that would benefit both growers and consumers is the greater ease with which they can be grown organically. Much of the pesticide used on leaf crops is to ensure the visual perfection demanded by consumers. This cosmetic use of pesticides could be dropped because the leaves will be ground to a fine powder before the customer sees them. This could move leaf vegetables out of the "dirty dozen" category of foods most likely to have pesticide residue.

This is a move that most consumers—even those who don't currently buy organic produce—would welcome. In addition, drying leafy vegetables can reduce the risk of food poisoning. Quickly heating leaf vegetables before drying reduces bacteria count nearly 100 percent. This would have eliminated the *E. coli* on spinach that sickened hundreds of people—and killed three—in the US in the fall of 2006.

Leaf powders could be integrated into the diets of young children and the elderly. These are people who often find the tough or stringy texture of greens to be a struggle for their limited dental resources. Children under five years old are in the most critical period of their growth, when good nutrition is most vital. The elderly are the fastest-growing segment of the human population and they are uniquely vulnerable to many diet-related health problems. Making greens more useful and acceptable to these two groups is an important undertaking.

It is already possible to buy dried leaf powder on the Internet. (Several sources are listed in Appendix 1.) Spinach powder is commonly available at a reasonable price from food ingredient suppliers, since it is used in spinach pasta and dips. Green onion and parsley flakes are widely available in bulk, as are many other leaves normally used for seasoning. Moringa leaf powder is now being offered through several outlets. Kale powder and powder from wheat and barley leaves are being sold, but mainly as high-priced supplements through alternative health sites. It is still quite unusual to find dried leaf powders in ordinary retail food shops.

By extending shelf life, reducing weight and volume, and eliminating much of the risk of pesticide and microorganism contamination, drying leaf crops creates some new possibilities for eating more greens. Fine grinding removes most of the texture problems that have restrained use of greens, especially among children and the elderly. The versatility of solar-dried green leaf powder enables it to be used in countless foods that have traditionally been outside the realm of leaf vegetables.

13

Making Both Ends Meat

❊ ❊ ❊

Concentrating the Nutrition of Green Leaves

As hunters and gatherers, humans grew up understanding the value of meat. Though the gathering may have paid most of the bills, meat had special significance both nutritionally and culturally. We sought after meat because game animals predigest and concentrate the nutrients from the plants they eat, making the nutrients in meat both abundant and easily absorbed. This combination has made meat almost universally desirable as a food.

We've never lost our appetite for meat. Meat is too expensive for the people occupying the lower rungs of life's ladder, but as we grow wealthier we eat more meat. Chinese meat consumption, for example, has increased about five-fold as their economy has strengthened over the past 20 years. Similar increases in meat eating are taking place in India, Brazil, Mexico, and other rapidly developing countries—though they still lag well behind the wealthier, more carnivorous societies of North America, Europe, and Australia.

Adding a small amount of meat to the diet of people living on a few dollars (or less) a day would provide them with a significant health benefit. It could supply high-quality protein and readily usable iron, vitamin A, zinc, and other essential nutrients missing from the starchy staples that make up the bulk of the diet of the poor. Most North Americans no longer need such a high-octane nutritional package. For us, increased consumption of meat, especially red meat, has myriad negative health impacts, including increased risk of heart disease, colon and pancreatic cancer, osteoporosis, diabetes, kidney disease, hypertension, and obesity.

Our ancestral appetite for meat is also causing some major environmental damage. Loss of rain forest, soil erosion, greenhouse gases, pollution of surface water, and antibiotic-resistant bacteria are some of the environmental problems aggravated by increased meat production. Meat makes ecological sense when ruminants like cows and sheep are raised on coarse forage that they can convert into a smaller amount of more nutritionally dense food. It *doesn't* make sense when animals are fed cultivated corn and soy that could feed people directly. Meat is desirable, expensive, and hard on the environment.

Culturally, the hunting and sharing of game meat was an important ritual that strengthened the bonds of community. For most of us, the thrill of the hunt is long gone. The intrepid hunter has been replaced by a chump holding a can of lighter fluid and grilling in a "Kiss the Cook" apron. Still, the cultural status of meat remains high. Feeding the nine billion plus people expected at the global dinner table by 2050 without trashing the natural environment will be a Herculean undertaking, one made even more daunting as demand for meat increases.

One approach to this quandary has been to look for ways to make synthetic meat. This strategy took a big step forward in August 2013, when a laboratory-made hamburger was served up in London. The burger began as stem cells extracted during a biopsy of two cows. Like most people, you probably lack the resources to extract bovine stem cells (or the backyard to graze a few head of cattle).

However, you can still convert the foliage in your back yard into a super-nutritious food for your human family. A relatively simple process called *leaf fractionation* can mechanically separate the indigestible cellulose and create *leaf concentrate*, a plant-based food with meat-like nutritional attributes. While not much of a threat to steak houses or hamburger joints (at least for now), leaf concentration is potentially a powerful food technology that could become important as the natural world strains under the burden of feeding so many.

Though very few people have ever tasted leaf concentrate, it is not a new food technology. A Frenchman named Hilaire Marin Rouelle (1718–1779) made curd from green leaves over 200 years ago. He tried mashing the leaves of several types of crops with a marble mortar and pestle. He then strained out the leaf juice and heated it. Just before the leaf juice began to boil, a green curd formed and floated to the top. Almost all of the cellulose from the leaf cell walls and most of the water in the leaves were removed in this simple process. When as much liquid as is practical is pressed from this green curd, it is called *leaf concentrate* (or sometimes *leaf protein*, or even *leaf protein concentrate*). This pressed curd can then be dried to make a powder that is a truly remarkable food as the chart below illustrates.

Table 3. Nutrients in Selected High Protein Foods

100 g (3½ oz) edible portion	Protein (g)	Iron (mg)	Calcium (mg)	Vitamin A (mcg RAE)
Dried alfalfa leaf concentrate	50.8	54.0	3380.0	3835.0
Beef steak	29.0	1.9	22.0	0.0
Scrambled eggs	15.0	2.1	66.0	182.0
Dried whole milk	26.3	0.5	912.0	257.0
Dry pinto beans	21.4	5.1	113.0	0.0

Leaf concentrate composition from E. Bertin (2009). Composition nutritionelle detailée de l'extrait foliaire de luzerne (EFL). Association pour la Promotion des Extraits Foliaires en Nutrition. All others from USDA.

Economics favor making leaf concentrate on a scale large enough to justify specialized equipment, but it can certainly be made on a household scale using familiar kitchen equipment. The steps to making leaf concentrate are similar at every scale, from commercial operations (such as France Luzerne's in Aulnay, France, that processes 150 tons of alfalfa per hour) to peasants pounding leaves with wooden sticks.

Leaves are harvested, then rinsed in clean water as soon as possible. Then they are ground or pulped, which breaks open the leaf cell walls and liberates nutrients. Then the pulp is pressed to separate the leaf juice from the fiber. The green leaf juice is then heated quickly to the boiling point. Heat causes proteins and oils in the leaf to form a curd that floats to the top. This green curd is skimmed off and then pressed to remove as much liquid as possible. The moist leaf curd—leaf concentrate—can be eaten directly or dried and ground for later use.

As with all food processing, quality control throughout is critical. Burnt curd, leaf or curd spoilage, and inadequate pressing of the whey can all lead to leaf concentrate with unacceptable flavor.

Steps for Making Leaf Concentrate at Home

1. Harvest fresh green leaves. Not all edible leaves make good leaf concentrate. Legumes, such as cowpeas and alfalfa, and tender young grasses are the best. Avoid leaves that are sour (i.e., sorrel or roselle) or mucilaginous (i.e., vine spinach or jute).
2. Rinse the leaves to remove dust and dirt.
3. Cut the leaves into pieces the length of a finger.
4. Grind the leaves to a pulp in a blender or meat grinder.

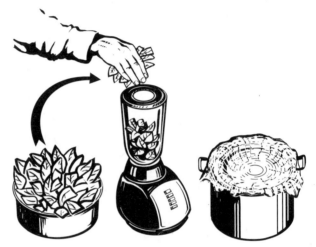

Grind leaves in blender.

5. Squeeze the juice from the leaf pulp as thoroughly as possible.

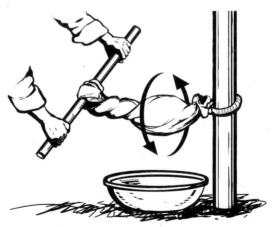

Wring juice from pulped leaves (can also be used to wring whey from leaf curd).

6. Heat the juice rapidly to the boiling point.
7. Separate the curd that forms in the heated juice and place in a tightly woven cloth.

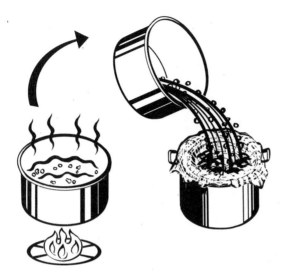

Separate the leaf curd by pouring the
liquid through a strong cloth.

8. Squeeze the liquid ("whey") from this curd as thoroughly as possible after it cools. What remains in the cloth is *leaf concentrate*.

Tips for Making Leaf Concentrate at Home

Leaves yield the most leaf concentrate just before the plants flower. Harvest crops for leaf concentrate in the morning when moisture content is high. Do not use a rotary lawn mower, as it will suck dust and dirt into the chopped leaves that is then impossible to remove.

Grind the leaves to a pulp as soon as possible after harvesting. I repeat: *Don't delay grinding after harvesting*. Yield will decline by about 15 percent in four hours and about 50 percent in nine hours. Flavor also suffers. You are trying to break open as many leaf cells as possible. As leaves wilt, the pressure inside the cells declines and the amount of force required to rupture the cell wall increases. A mildly entertaining visualization demonstrates this principle. Picture the cell as a water balloon. It is harder to burst when half full (wilted) than when completely filled with liquid (freshly harvested).

High-powered household blenders do a good job making small amounts of leaf concentrate. But any blender with less than 600 watts will likely burn out quickly from making leaf concentrate. (Wattage is usually posted on the bottom of the blender base.) Home-scale meat grinders also work for pulping leaves. Look for #22 and #32 meat grinders in sporting goods or hardware stores. They are sold to hunters for grinding up deer meat. It takes a little practice to get the hang of pulping leaves with a meat grinder, and it is usually messy. Consider it to be either hard work or good exercise. For making a small amount of leaf concentrate at home, try a blender first because it is the simplest in terms of machinery.

Separating the leaf juice from the indigestible fiber can be done by squeezing it through a strong nylon mesh found at any fabric store or the mesh bags sold at paint stores for straining paint. There are many ways to apply the pressure. Working with small quantities, I prefer using an extremely simple press made from the legs of blue jeans from secondhand stores. Other material, such as muslin, will work fine, but use fabric strong enough to hold up to repeated and vigorous wringing. It is a variation on the old fashioned wringing post that was used to wring water from clothes before they were hung to dry. You can add to the pressure being applied by using a broomstick to help twist the cloth.

Heat the leaf juice rapidly just to the point of reaching a full boil. This coagulates the leaf curd, kills most pathogens, and neutralizes enzymes that can cause bad flavor during storage. Gently scraping across the bottom of the cook pot a few times just before the juice reaches the boiling point will reduce the risk of burning the curd. Small amounts of leaf juice can be heated in a microwave oven to make curd. It is best to use heatproof glass rather than plastic containers.

Let the liquid cool before separating the curd to reduce the chance of being scalded. Pour the contents of the cook pot gradually through a filter cloth set inside a colander (the same type used for pasta). Then, remove the curd from the filter cloth and place the curd in a strong cloth (like denim) and press to remove as much of the whey as possible. This process is the same as pressing the juice from the fiber, except the pressure should be applied a bit more gradually and held for a longer time. The wringing pole approach works well for this step as well. After being pressed, the curd should be crumbly (about 60 percent moisture). You can determine the moisture content by weighing the fresh leaf curd then drying it thoroughly and dividing the dry weight by the fresh weight. For home use, though, "crumbly" is normally an adequate measure.

How to Use Leaf Concentrate

Replacing ten percent of the flour called for in recipes with leaf concentrate can pump up the nutrition in baked breads, cakes, crackers, and cookies. Many ethnic foods such as tamales, tortillas, chapattis, and pirogies can also be spiked with leaf concentrate. Because fresh leaf concentrate disperses more readily in liquids than does dried concentrate or dried leaves, it is easier to incorporate into a variety of soups, stews, sauces, and smoothies. A surprisingly refreshing green lemonade can be made by mixing two tablespoons of leaf concentrate lemon syrup (see Chapter 14 for recipe) in an eight-ounce glass of cold water. While it still contains a lot of sugar, it is far healthier than regular lemonade or soda.

If you enjoy playing in the kitchen, homemade pasta is another excellent way to use leaf concentrate. Replacing ten percent of the flour in any pasta recipe with leaf curd will kick it up to a much higher nutritional level. Children who refuse to eat vegetables are often happy to eat green pasta. It can be made with fresh or dried leaf concentrate, and the pasta itself can then be used immediately or dried for later use. Instructions for making the green leaf-enriched pasta is in the recipe section in Chapter 14.

Drying Leaf Concentrate

Fresh leaf concentrate will last a week to ten days in a sealed container in the refrigerator. However, there are some advantages to preserving it for later use. Leaves tend to be more plentiful at certain times and may be completely unavailable over long winters or dry seasons. Drying leaf concentrate lets you turn a temporary surplus of fresh leaves into a year-round supply of high-nutrition food. Also, bear in mind that making leaf concentrate is a big mess. The amount of work required getting set up and then cleaning up is about the same regardless of how much leaf curd is produced. This, too, argues for making larger batches less frequently and finding a way to preserve the product for later use.

The best way to preserve leaf concentrate is to dry it to below ten percent moisture. This is too little moisture for spoilage microbes to reproduce. Fully dried leaf concentrate can be stored for up to a year if kept cool in an airtight container and out of the light. Dried leaf concentrate will retain its qualities even better if stored in a refrigerator or freezer.

Drying leaf concentrate is very similar to drying fresh green leaves. Almost all of the information on drying leaf vegetables in Chapter 12 applies to drying leaf concentrate as well. There are many electric food dryers for sale, and the solar leaf dryer described in Chapter 12 works well with leaf concentrate. It is inexpensive, easy to build, and has no fuel costs. As with leaves, leaf concentrate should be completely dried in one day. It will dry faster and more evenly if the curd is pushed through a ¼" mesh to granulate it before drying.

Leaf concentrate can be also preserved by freezing it in a tightly sealed freezer bag. Once it is thawed, it can be used in any of the ways that the fresh product is used, though the texture is altered somewhat. Other methods of preserving, such as pickling, fermenting, and canning have been less well developed and probably don't bring much advantage.

Table 4. Leaf Concentrate Math

Approximate yield from 4.5 pounds (2 kilograms) of fresh leaves	
Leaf concentrate (fresh)	3½ ounces (100 grams) @ 50–60% water content
or	
Leaf concentrate (dried)	1½ ounces (40 grams) @ 7–10% water content
plus	
Whey	1 quart (1 liter) @ 93–98% water content
Fibre	2¼ lbs (1 kilogram) @ 50–60% water content

A typical serving is about an ounce of fresh leaf concentrate or one-third of an ounce of dried. Four and a half pounds of fresh leaves should yield about four servings.

Removing the stems can nearly double the percentage yield of leaf concentrate. For instance, 100 pounds of a forage variety of cowpeas, such as Iron and Clay, will yield about 2 pounds of dried leaf concentrate. You will get roughly the same 2 pounds if you remove the leaves from the stems before grinding them. There will be about 55 pounds of leaf and 45 pounds of stem.

Stripping leaves from their stems reduces by nearly half how much grinding, pressing, and heating must be done per pound of leaf concentrate. Of course, it adds the labor of stripping the leaves.

Two crops of cowpeas in a fertile 100-square-foot garden bed should be able to produce 100 servings of leaf concentrate in a year. Cowpeas are fast, easy to grow, and drought tolerant. Seed is cheap and the inoculant for fixing nitrogen is readily available. Happily, there are a number of other crops that are almost as good as cowpeas. Although the yields of leaf crops vary greatly with climate, soil, variety, planting density, and cultivation techniques, alfalfa, hyacinth beans, winter peas, wheat, and barley are among the crops that can produce leaf concentrate at this level.

Using the Whole Plant

The leaf concentrate makes up less than five percent of the total weight of the plant. After the leaf concentrate is separated from the plant, there still remains the roots and stems in addition to the residual fiber and whey. Making good use of the other parts of the plant is essential to making leaf concentrate economically viable.

Plant roots will break down and feed the soil without any human intervention. So leaving them in place when you harvest is a good idea. Stems and residual fiber can be used to improve garden soil or as animal feed for cattle, horses, sheep, goats, and rabbits (though probably too calcium-rich to be a good choice as a primary feed for rabbits over six months old). Chickens and pigs will often eat the fiber but, like us, they are unable to digest the cellulose, so they derive little value from it. Usually, it takes animals a few days to a couple of weeks to get used to this new feed.

For kitchen gardeners, the best use of the stems and fiber left from making leaf concentrate is usually the simplest: returning it to the garden as mulch or compost. These leftovers make excellent mulch that adds nutrients, feeds beneficial soil organisms, conserves soil moisture, and reduces competition from weeds. It should not be applied in layers over two inches thick, or it can form a mat that

Feed leftover fiber to goats, cows, sheep, horses, or rabbits.

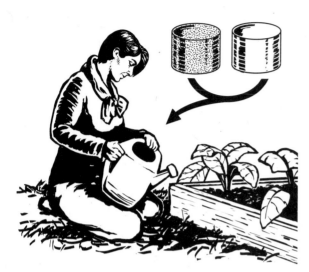

Mix whey with an equal amount of water and use to irrigate garden.

water doesn't easily penetrate. It can, however, be added to compost piles in fairly thick layers and will quickly break down into a useful product for improving soil structure.

The liquid, or whey, remaining from making leaf concentrate can be re-mixed with the fiber and fed to animals, or it can be diluted with an equal volume of water and sprinkled on your garden. The whey contains enough nitrogen and potassium to be valuable as a liquid fertilizer.

In Chapter 11, alfalfa, cowpeas, winter peas, wheat, and barley were noted as being among the best of the edible soil-improving cover crops. They are also among the top crops for making leaf concentrate. Combining an edible cover crop with leaf concentrate production creates a powerful synergy that can provide important nutritional, agricultural, and economic benefits. In theory, you could even develop a lawn based on edible grasses and legumes that could be periodically harvested to make leaf concentrate.

Leaf Concentrate in Perspective

Much of the early research on leaf concentrate took place in England. Originally, it was viewed as an alternative source of protein during World War II, when food supplies were interrupted on that island nation. When the war ended and food imports began flowing freely again, interest in leaf concentrate waned. It has reappeared again mainly as a tool to fight serious malnutrition in the tropics.

For seriously malnourished children, leaf concentrate is a life saver. For people suffering AIDS or other health problems that affect their ability to eat and digest food, it has been extremely valuable. The very high nutrient-to-weight ratio of dried leaf concentrate makes it a promising emergency food to ship into disaster areas and refugee camps that don't have a functioning food system.

But what about the average well-nourished home gardener? Leaf concentrate can certainly be made on a home-kitchen scale, and it is a fascinating thing to try making at least once. It is instructive in understanding how our food is formed in the green leaves of plants and how the little cardboard-like boxes that make up plant cell walls prevent us from accessing much of that food value.

However, like eating meat every day, eating leaf concentrate is not something most North Americans need to do. It may be useful for vegans and vegetarians who abstain from eating meat. Women who are vegetarians are especially susceptible to iron deficiency anemia because of menstruation, and they may profit from the high bio-availability of the iron in leaf concentrate. People prone to forming painful calcium oxalate kidney stones are often told to avoid green leafy vegetables. Because the soluble oxalic acid is removed from leaves during the process, leaf concentrate is usually safe for them to eat. Children who refuse to eat vegetables—a sizable and vocal group—may benefit from such a concentrated and well-disguised source of veggies. People who are sick, recovering from illness, elderly, or just need a nutritional boost may all find leaf concentrate useful.

Leaf concentrate is a remarkable food with great potential. It is far easier to make and less ethically complicated than lab-cultured bovine burgers. I'm surprised the late-night telemarketers haven't seized upon it yet.

Leaf Concentrate: A Field Guide for Small-scale Programs is a useful guide for people seriously interested in working with this food. It is available in both English and Spanish at leafforlife.org.

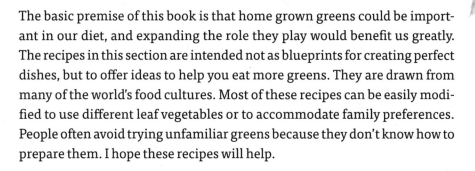

14

Recipes

❅ ❅ ❅

From the Garden to the Table

The basic premise of this book is that home grown greens could be important in our diet, and expanding the role they play would benefit us greatly. The recipes in this section are intended not as blueprints for creating perfect dishes, but to offer ideas to help you eat more greens. They are drawn from many of the world's food cultures. Most of these recipes can be easily modified to use different leaf vegetables or to accommodate family preferences. People often avoid trying unfamiliar greens because they don't know how to prepare them. I hope these recipes will help.

Soups

Cream of Chaya Soup

Red Callaloo

Roasted Vegetables and Kale Soup

Spicy Jute (Molokhia) Leaf Soup

Salads

Kale Salad with Tahini Dressing

Orzo Salad with Wild Greens
    and Feta

Sweet Potato Leaves Salad

Tabouli

Dishes with Cooked Greens

Amaranth Leaves with Black Beans

Bitter Gourd Leaf and Moringa Leaf
    Vegetable Stew

Carrot-Wolfberry Leaf Stir-Fry

Cheesy Grits with Okinawa Spinach

Green Mexican Tamales

Green Pasta

Lentil Stew with Roselle Leaves

Pumpkin Leaf with Peanuts
Quail Grass Tomato Basil Quiche

Saag Paneer

Snacks/ Sauces/Drinks/Others

Dinosaur Cookies
Green Birthday Cake
Green Gomasio (Gomashio)
Green Smoothie
Kale Chips
Kimchi

Leaf Concentrate Lemonade Syrup
Malabar Bars
Power Balls
Shiso Pesto
Stuffed Grape Leaves

Cream of Chaya Soup

Ingredients:

2 cups packed chaya leaves, washed, stems removed, and chopped into small pieces

1 garlic clove, crushed

1 small onion, chopped

1 cup of vegetable broth

4 fresh basil leaves, chopped, or 1 tsp dried basil

2 cups milk

salt and pepper to taste

red chili pepper

yogurt or unsweetened cream

Directions:

Put chopped chaya leaves, garlic, onion, and vegetable broth in a pot and cook 10–15 minutes until the leaves are softened.

Add milk and basil.

Blend in a blender until all ingredients are well mixed.

Return to pot, add salt and pepper to taste. Heat slowly until very hot, being careful not to let it boil.

Serve in bowls. For a final touch, add a tablespoon or more of yogurt or unsweetened cream to the middle. Optional: sprinkle with crushed red chili peppers.

Makes 4 cups.

Red Callaloo

Callaloo is a classic leaf-based soup or stew from the Caribbean, with as many variations as there are islands. Amaranth leaves, taioba, and taro leaves are three of the favorites. Soup captures water-soluble vitamins that are often lost when leaves are boiled. This soup is rich in nutrients and is especially good for losing weight because it is filling, but low in calories.

Ingredients:

1 cup red amaranth leaves, chopped

1 cup chaya or taioba leaves, chopped

1 small onion, finely chopped

1 tomato, chopped

½ cup okra, sliced

2 garlic cloves, crushed

1 tsp fresh thyme, finely chopped

1 cup water or broth

1 cup coconut milk

½ tsp chili sauce

salt to taste

Directions:

Put all ingredients in pot. Bring to near boiling, then simmer for 45 minutes.

Serves 4.

soup

Roasted Vegetables and Kale Soup

Ingredients:

4 cups of root vegetables (such as turnips, sweet potatoes, carrots, white potatoes, rutabaga, and beets). Use any combination that equals 4 cups.

2 large tomatoes

1 large onion

1–2 Tbs olive oil

salt and pepper

6 garlic cloves

6–7 cups vegetable broth

4 cups kale, washed, stemmed, and chopped coarsely

1 Tbs fresh thyme

1 bay leaf

1 can (15 oz) great white northern beans, drained

Directions:

Preheat oven to 400 degrees.

Wash and cut all root vegetables into small bite-sized pieces. Drizzle a baking sheet with olive oil and place vegetables on top. Drizzle more olive oil on top of vegetables and sprinkle with salt and pepper.

Wash and cut tomatoes into quarters. Peel onion and cut into 6 wedges. Take a second baking sheet, drizzle with oil, and put tomatoes and onions on it, drizzling more oil on top. Sprinkle with salt and pepper.

Place both baking sheets in the oven. Bake until the root vegetables are tender, about 40 minutes. Stir occasionally.

When done, peel garlic and place in a food processor with the onions and tomatoes. Add ½ cup of vegetable broth and puree until smooth.

Transfer into a large pot and add remaining vegetable broth, the kale, thyme, and bay leaf. Bring to a boil then simmer until the kale is cooked, about 20 minutes.

Add the roasted root vegetables and the beans, and simmer for a few minutes to meld flavors. If needed, add more vegetable broth. Adjust seasonings and serve.

Can be made a day ahead.

Serves 4–6.

Spicy Jute (Molokhia) Leaf Soup

Ingredients:

2 cups fresh jute (molokhia) leaves
(may use frozen leaves if fresh is
not available)
6 cups chicken or vegetable broth
2 hot chili peppers, minced
1 bay leaf
¾ cup onion, diced
black pepper to taste

1½ tsp garlic, minced
1 tsp ground coriander
1 tsp olive oil
½ lb tofu, cut into bite-size pieces
(optional)
2 Tbs fresh cilantro, chopped
1 Tbs lemon juice
cayenne pepper to taste

Directions:

Chop molokhia leaves into strips. Set aside.

In large pot, heat the vegetable broth. Add molokhia leaves, chili pepper, bay leaf, onion, and black pepper. Stir. Reduce heat and let simmer.

Mash garlic and coriander into a paste. In small fry pan, sauté garlic paste and tofu chunks (if using) in olive oil until garlic is slightly browned. Add to the soup and stir.

After soup has simmered for about 20–30 minutes, add the cilantro, lemon juice, and cayenne pepper. Stir and let simmer for another 5 minutes.

Serve hot over rice or "as is" with slices of good crusty bread on the side.

Serves 4–6.

Kale Salad with Tahini Dressing

Ingredients:

4 packed cups of kale, washed, stemmed, and chopped

½ cup lemon juice

½ cup olive oil

2 Tbs tahini

2 Tbs soy sauce

3 cloves garlic, crushed

¼ tsp honey (optional)

Optional additions:

1 cup grated carrots

2 cups roasted white potatoes, in 1-inch pieces

2 cups roasted sweet potatoes, in 1-inch pieces

¼ cup dried cranberries or raisins

½ cup nuts (pine nuts, walnuts, or almonds are good possibilities)

1 orange, segmented and cut into bite-size pieces

Directions:

Place chopped kale in a large bowl. Add any of the optional additions in any combination that sounds good.

In a separate bowl, whisk together lemon juice, olive oil, tahini, soy sauce, crushed garlic, and honey.

Pour half of the dressing onto the kale salad using your clean hands to massage the dressing well into the kale. Continue adding more dressing as needed to fully coat the leaves.

Let stand for 20–30 minutes before serving.

Serves 4–6.

Orzo Salad with Wild Greens and Feta

Orzo is a small pasta. Quinoa may replace the orzo if you are looking for a gluten-free dish.

Ingredients:

½ lb orzo

4 cups of greens; any combination of dandelion greens, pigweed, or plantain greens washed, stemmed, and chopped.

¾ cup walnuts, chopped

¾ cup red onion, diced or thinly sliced

¾ cup feta cheese, crumbled

½ cup olive oil

2 garlic cloves

¼ tsp salt

½ tsp pepper

Directions:

Cook orzo until done, rinse under cool water, drain well, and put in a bowl.

In a separate pan, boil a small amount of water, add the greens and cook until tender.

Drain well and add to the orzo.

Add the walnuts, onion, and feta cheese.

Whisk together olive oil, garlic, salt and pepper. Pour over the orzo mixture and toss. Adjust seasonings and serve.

Serves 4.

Sweet Potato Leaves Salad

Ingredients:

2 cups water

2 cups sweet potato leaves (stems removed), washed, and chopped

12 cherry tomatoes, halved

1 small red onion, sliced finely

3 Tbs rice vinegar

1 tsp shredded ginger

½ tsp sugar

salt and pepper to taste

Directions:

Place water in cooking pot and bring to a boil. Blanch the sweet potato leaves by dropping them in the boiling water for about 30–45 seconds. Then drain the water, and put the leaves immediately in a cold water bath so they will cool quickly. Drain, and let leaves dry on a clean towel.

In a large bowl, combine the sweet potato leaves with the tomatoes and onion.

Whisk together the vinegar, ginger, sugar, salt and pepper, and toss lightly with the vegetables.

Serve immediately.

Yields 4 side salads.

Tabouli

Ingredients:

½ cup dry bulgur wheat
¾ cup boiling water
½ tsp salt
2 Tbs lemon or lime juice
2 cloves garlic, crushed

1–2 Tbs olive oil
¾ cup fresh parsley, chopped
¼ cup green onions, chopped
1 tomato, diced

Directions:

Combine bulgur, salt, and boiling water in bowl. Cover and let sit until all the water is absorbed.

Add lemon juice, garlic, and olive oil; mix thoroughly. Let marinate for 2–3 hours in refrigerator.

Add parsley, onions, and tomato. Mix gently and serve.

Serves 2–3.

Amaranth Leaves with Black Beans

This is a very easy recipe where amaranth greens are simply added to flavored beans. There are, of course, many variations of this by simply changing the type of beans, the type of greens, or the flavorings.

Ingredients:

1 medium onion, chopped finely

2 garlic cloves, crushed

1 can of black beans with juice or
   2 cups of cooked black beans

4 Tbs cilantro, chopped

salt and hot sauce to taste

2 scant cups of amaranth, washed,
   stemmed, and well chopped

Directions:

Sauté chopped onion and garlic in a small amount of oil. When onion is translucent, add the beans with bean juice, cilantro, salt, and hot sauce. Simmer for about 20–30 minutes.

While the bean mixture is simmering, bring a pot with a little water to a boil and add the amaranth leaves. Blanch for 3 minutes, then drain.

Add to the beans, simmer for a few minutes, adjust seasonings, and serve.

This recipe can be served as is, put into tortillas, or served on top of rice.

Serves 4.

Bitter Gourd Leaf and Moringa Leaf Vegetable Stew

Although bitter gourd is widely popular in south Asia, it is, as the name implies, quite bitter and is often an acquired taste in western countries.

Ingredients:

2 tsp olive oil

2 cloves garlic, crushed

¼ cup onions, diced

½ cup fresh or canned tomatoes, diced

1½ cups water

1 cup of potato, cubed

1 large carrot, cubed

1 cup broccoli, chopped

1 small eggplant, thinly sliced

2 tsp red curry paste

1 Tbs lime juice

¾ cup moringa leaves, washed, stemmed, and chopped

⅓ cup young bitter gourd leaves, washed, stemmed, and chopped

salt and pepper to taste

Directions:

Sauté garlic and onion in olive oil in a large saucepan. When onion is transparent, add tomatoes, water, and potatoes. Boil for 5 minutes. Add carrots, broccoli, eggplant, red curry paste, and lime juice. Cook for 7 minutes more on medium heat. Toss in moringa and bitter gourd leaves, salt and pepper and cook until the leaves are softened, about 2–3 minutes. Stir often. If needed, add small amounts of water to keep the mixture moist. Adjust spices. Can be served as is or over rice.

Serves 2.

*dishes with
cooked greens*

Carrot-Wolfberry Leaf Stir-Fry

Ingredients:

5 cups of tender young wolfberry
 leaves, washed and chopped

3 Tbs olive oil

8 garlic cloves, crushed

1 lb tofu, cut into bite-size cubes

¾ cup scallions, chopped

1 cup carrots sliced into thin strips

3 Tbs finely grated fresh ginger

3 Tbs soy sauce

¼ tsp of black pepper

Directions:

Prepare leaves and set aside.

Heat oil and garlic in a pan on medium heat.

Toss in the tofu, scallions, carrots, and ginger. Cook for 3–5 minutes until cooked. Stir frequently to prevent sticking.

Add the soy sauce, pepper, and the wolfberry leaves, and continue cooking until leaves are soft. (About 2–3 minutes. Leaves cook quickly.)

Serve as a side dish or serve over rice, couscous, millet, or quinoa for a main dish.

Serves 4.

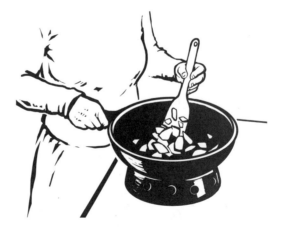

Stir-frying cooks leaf vegetables quickly
with little loss of nutrition.

Cheesy Grits with Okinawa Spinach

Ingredients:

1 cup coarsely chopped Okinawa
   spinach leaves
½ cup yellow grits
2¼ cups water

¼ tsp salt
margarine or butter (optional)
cheddar cheese
black pepper to taste

Directions:

Wash the Okinawa spinach, remove any large stems, and chop the leaves into small pieces.

Microwave or simmer the corn grits in salted water for about 2 minutes. While it is still soupy, add the Okinawa spinach and cook for another 3 minutes, or until the grits are firm.

Dish into bowls and top with a pat of butter or margarine, and/or a generous sprinkling of grated cheddar cheese and some black pepper.

Serves 4.

Green Mexican Tamales

*Making tamales is often an entertaining social event. Extra tamales can be
frozen for later use.*

Ingredients:

2 cups masa harina or cornmeal
⅓ cup dried leaf powder or leaf
    concentrate
2 tsp baking powder

1 tsp salt
⅓ cup vegetable shortening
1½ cups soup stock or water
dried corn leaves (around 24)

Directions:

Soak corn leaves in warm water for about 30 minutes until they become
flexible, then carefully separate them.

Combine dry ingredients.

Beat the shortening until creamy, then gradually beat in the dry ingredients. Slowly add the soup stock or water, stirring constantly.

Spread about 1 tablespoon of this dough in the center of a clean corn leaf.
Wrap the dough in the corn leaf by neatly folding in the edges. Repeat until
all the dough is wrapped.

Steam the tamales for 40–60 minutes. Serve hot. This makes around 24
tamales.

Serves 8–12.

Note: Chili or other flavorings and sweeteners can be added to the tamale
dough, or a teaspoon of cheese or meat can be placed on the center of the
dough before it is wrapped.

Green Pasta

Pasta was first eaten in China over 1,500 years ago. It has been gaining in popularity ever since. Everyone agrees that homemade pasta is the best, and pasta making is a fun activity for children! Replacing 20 percent of the flour with dried leaf powder or leaf concentrate turns a favorite food into a convenient dynamo of good nutrition.

Ingredients:

2 cups all-purpose or bread flour (½ semolina flour and ½ all-purpose flour is ideal)

½ tsp salt
½ cup dried green leaf powder or leaf concentrate
water

Directions:

Mix flour and salt, then add leaf powder or concentrate and a small amount of water. Knead for 10 minutes. Dough should be heavy, but elastic. Roll the dough out as thin as possible and cut into strips. If your dough is too wet, the strips will stick together; too dry and the pasta will break apart during cooking. The strips can be cooked fresh or dried in a dark room, sealed in a plastic bag, and cooked when convenient. This pasta cooks somewhat faster than commercial pasta.

Hand-operated stainless steel pasta rollers are available in some cook shops and over the Internet for about $40–$75. They make very uniform pasta. Machines made in Italy are

4 cups of flour to 1 cup of fine leaf powder.

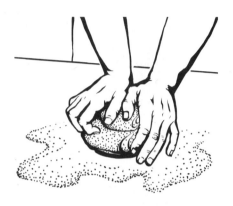

Knead pasta dough.

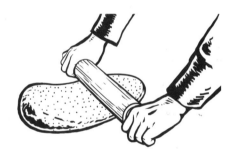

Roll out pasta dough with a rolling pin.

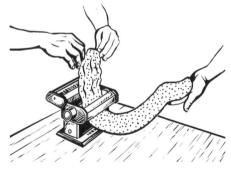

Feed dough through a hand-operated machine.

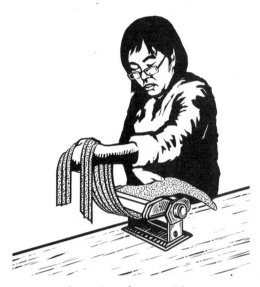

Cut strips of pasta with a
hand-operated machine.

generally the best quality. With some patience,
pasta can be made without a machine, but it is a
lot of work, and the results will be less uniform.

A simple variation is spaetzle. This is pasta
dough that is pushed through the largest-size
openings on a cheese grater. It is usually grated
directly into boiling water, hot broth, or soup,
where it cooks almost instantly and floats to
the top.

Serves 4–6.

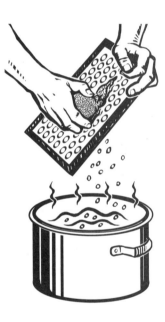

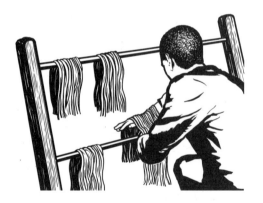

Hang pasta to dry on a simple rack.

Grating pasta dough into boiling
soup is a simple variation.

Lentil Stew with Roselle Leaves

Ingredients:

2 cups roselle leaves (cranberry hibiscus or okra leaves can substitute)

½ cup yellow peas

1½ cups water

1 tsp salt

2 Tbs olive oil

½ tsp cumin seed

½ tsp mustard seed

2 garlic cloves, crushed

¾ cup onion, chopped

½–1 tsp red curry paste

1¼ cups water

¼ tsp turmeric powder

Directions:

Wash roselle leaves, remove stems, chop into small pieces, and set aside.

Put yellow peas, 1½ cups of water, and salt in a sauce pan and simmer until peas are soft (about 30 minutes).

While the peas are cooking, take a separate pan, heat the oil, add the cumin seed, mustard seed, garlic, and onion, and cook until the onion is translucent. Stir frequently. If needed, add a small amount of water to prevent sticking.

When the onion is translucent, add the roselle leaves and the red curry paste and 1¼ cups of water.

Continue cooking until the leaves are soft (about 8 minutes).

Add the turmeric and the cooked yellow peas and continue cooking until water is cooked off and the desired consistency is reached (about 8 minutes).

Serve over rice, corn grits, couscous, quinoa, or a grain of your choice.

Serves 4.

Pumpkin Leaf and Peanut

This is an important dish in much of sub-Saharan Africa. A popular variation on this is the Congolese dish saka-saka, made with cassava leaves and peanut butter. Any hearty leaf vegetable such as walking stick kale, collards, or young cowpea leaves can substitute for the pumpkin leaf.

Ingredients:

1 Tbs vegetable oil

3 cups fresh pumpkin leaves, chopped

1 medium tomato, diced

1 cup finely chopped peanuts or ½ cup peanut butter

2½ cups water

salt and chili to taste

Directions:

Heat oil in large skillet. When hot, add pumpkin leaves and tomato. When leaves are tender, add peanuts. Slowly add water and spices, stirring constantly until a creamy paste is formed.

Serve over rice, couscous, bulgur, or pasta.

Serves 4.

Quail Grass Tomato Basil Quiche

Ingredients:

10-inch pie crust

1 cup onion or scallions, chopped

1–2 Tbs olive oil

4 very large tomatoes, chopped into bite-size pieces

1–1½ cups potatoes, washed and shredded

6 large eggs

1 cup milk

2 Tbs flour

1–2 garlic cloves, minced

¼ tsp salt

pepper to taste

4 oz sharp cheddar cheese

¾ cup quail grass leaves, washed, stemmed, and chopped into small pieces (amaranth or spinach can substitute)

½ cup basil leaves, washed, stemmed, and chopped finely

Directions:

Lay crust out in a pie plate. Set in the refrigerator to chill while preparing the quiche.

Sauté the onions in the oil. After 1–2 minutes, add the tomatoes, and continue cooking just until the onions are translucent. Add a dash of salt and pepper. Set aside in a separate bowl.

Use the same pan to fry the potatoes, adding a bit more oil so the potatoes will not stick. Cook until they are lightly browned. Set aside.

In a bowl, make a custard by beating together the eggs, milk, flour, garlic, salt, pepper, and half the cheese.

To assemble the quiche: Layer the onions and tomatoes on the crust. Put the quail grass and half the basil leaves on top of this followed by the potatoes. Pour the egg mixture over all of this.

Sprinkle the remaining cheese and basil on top.

Bake in a pre-heated oven at 375 degrees for about 45 minutes or until the center is solid.

Serves 4–6.

Saag Paneer

Ingredients:

2 lb fresh spinach, washed and
  trimmed
¼ cup vegetable oil
½ lb cubed fresh mozzarella or
  firm tofu
1 yellow onion, finely chopped

3 garlic cloves, minced
1 tsp freshly grated ginger
2 tsp curry powder
½ cup buttermilk
¼ cup plain yogurt
salt

Directions:

Bring a small amount of water to a boil, toss in the spinach, and cook for
1 minute. Drain the spinach well. Chop finely.

Heat the oil in a deep skillet on medium-high. Add the cubed cheese or
tofu and fry for a couple of minutes until light brown on all sides, gently
turning to avoid breaking up the cubes. Remove from skillet and set aside.

Return the skillet to the heat and sauté the onion, garlic, and ginger. Cook
about 5 minutes until soft, stirring occasionally. Add curry powder, and
cook for another minute, then add chopped spinach. Remove from heat
and stir in buttermilk, yogurt, and salt. The mixture should be thick and
creamy. Gently add cheese or tofu.

Serve with rice or chapatis.

Serves 4.

Dinosaur Cookies

These are a great way to trick innocent children into eating leafy green vegetables. Kids who would need to be forced to eat a serving of turnip greens will fight over who gets a stegosaurus cookie with a yellow eye. You might also try cookies shaped like frogs, turtles, alligators, clover, or Christmas trees—anything that makes a recognizable shape that is normally green.

Ingredients:

1⅔ cup flour	¾ cup butter or margarine
⅓ cup dried leaf powder or leaf concentrate	¾ cup sugar
	1 egg
¼ tsp salt	1 tsp almond extract

Directions:

Preheat oven to 325 degrees. Combine flour, leaf powder, and salt. Beat butter and sugar until creamy in a separate bowl. Add egg and flavoring. Beat well. Add flour mixture.

Gather dough into a ball. Refrigerate 1 hour, then roll dough until ¼-inch thick. Cut out shapes and add candy eyes if desired.

Bake 13–15 minutes. Do not brown.

Yields about 36 cookies.

Green Birthday Cake

This cake is best made with mild-flavored dried greens. Leaves of wheat, barley, cowpeas, or Austrian winter peas are ideal. These leaves are great edible cover crops as well.

Ingredients:

1 cup all-purpose flour
¼ cup finely ground dried green
   leaf powder
⅔ cup sugar
2 tsp baking powder

¼ cup butter or margarine, softened
⅔ cup milk
1 egg
2 tsp vanilla or almond flavoring

Directions:

In a bowl, combine flour, leaf powder, sugar, and baking powder.

Add the butter or margarine, milk, egg, and flavoring. Mix ingredients, then beat vigorously until batter is very smooth (1 minute on medium speed with electric beater).

Pour into an 8-inch round greased and floured baking pan.

Bake in oven at 350 degrees for 25–30 minutes until a toothpick inserted into the middle comes out clean. Let cool 5 minutes before removing from pan.

Serves 6–8.

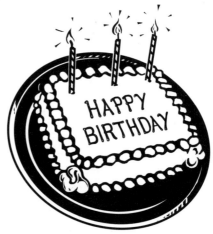

Leaf enriched birthday cake

Green Gomasio (Gomashio)

Sprinkle over rice, potatoes, or popcorn as an alternative to salt.

Ingredients:
1 cup raw brown sesame seeds
½ Tbs salt

½ Tbs dried Toon leaf, very finely ground

Directions:
Toast sesame seeds and salt over a medium flame until the seeds begin to pop open. Mix in dried leaf powder. Lightly grind in a coffee mill or a mortar and pestle. Most of the seeds should be cracked open but not ground into a paste.

Green Smoothie

Ingredients:
2 cups of spinach, kale, Swiss chard, parsley, or vine spinach, washed, stemmed, and ripped into large pieces.
2 cups of water

1 cup of mango or blueberries or raspberries
1 cup of pineapple
2 bananas

Directions:
Put the greens and the water in a blender and blend well. Add the other ingredients and blend until smooth. Pour into 2 glasses and enjoy.

Serves 2.

Some tips for making green smoothies:
To get a really velvety smoothie, blend greens in the water (or other liquid) first, and then add the fruits or other vegetables.

Bananas help thicken the smoothie, offering a nice consistency. If you don't like bananas, try freezing them first to reduce flavor or simply don't use them. Pick another fruit instead.

Add at least one frozen fruit so the smoothie will be cold.

There are endless variations on the smoothie idea, and it is fun to try new ones by using ingredients that you have on hand. They all can be made more nutritious by adding green leafy vegetables.

Check out the website simplegreensmoothies.com for tips, examples, and more recipe ideas.

Kale Chips

Serve these as a snack or appetizer.

Ingredients:

6–8 cups of kale (curly, lacinato, or red Russian all work well)

1–2 Tbs of oil (olive, sesame, or avocado oil all work well)

salt or seasoned salt

Directions:

Preheat oven to 350 degrees.

Wash kale, remove big stems, and dry well either on a clean towel or in a spinner.

Put the leaves in a large bowl and toss lightly with the oil.

Lay them in a single layer on a baking sheet. You may need two baking sheets.

Bake until they are crisp but not burned, (about 15 minutes) turning them once about half way through the baking time.

Sprinkle with salt or with seasoned salt when they come out of the oven.

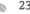

Kimchi

Ingredients:

1 lb red and/or green cabbage,
    shredded
1 large carrot, sliced thinly
2 scallions, sliced thinly
¼ cup soy sauce
½ cup water

2 Tbs honey
3 Tbs apple cider vinegar
1 tsp fresh ginger, minced
4 cloves garlic
2–4 dried small hot peppers,
    cut lengthwise

Directions:

Put shredded cabbage, carrots, and scallion in a bowl. Toss with soy sauce and water. Cover and let stand overnight.

Drain liquid from vegetables into a bowl. Add honey and vinegar to the drained liquid and stir well. Add ginger, garlic, and peppers to the vegetables, and pack them into a sterilized, 1-quart canning jar. Pour the liquid into the jar. If more liquid is needed to cover vegetables, add water. Cover loosely with a lid and let sit for 3–5 days to ferment. The liquid will bubble and the flavor will become sour. Kimchi should then be refrigerated. In 3 more days it can be served, or it can be stored in a refrigerator for 2 months.

Yields 1 quart.

Leaf Concentrate Lemonade Syrup

Ingredients:

1 cup lemon juice

½ cup fresh, well pressed leaf
   concentrate

1½ cups sugar

Directions:

Put lemon juice in a blender, add leaf concentrate, and blend well at highest speed. Gradually add sugar until all three ingredients are thoroughly blended. This makes about 1 pint of syrup.

The whole pint of syrup can be mixed with a gallon of water to make a nutritious lemonade. One glass of lemonade can be made by mixing two tablespoons of the syrup into 8 ounces of water. It should be used within a few days or refrigerated. The recipe can be adjusted to taste. It is especially good for anyone with anemia.

Yields 16 glasses.

Malabar Bars

Quail grass, amaranth, spinach, Swiss chard, or other mild-flavored greens can be substituted for vine spinach. These bars make delicious and nourishing mid-morning or after-school snacks.

Ingredients:

3 eggs
1 cup flour
1 cup skim milk
1 tsp salt
1 tsp baking powder

½ lb sharp cheddar cheese, grated
1 small onion, chopped finely
2 cups cooked, chopped vine spinach leaves (also called Malabar spinach), well drained.

Directions:

Mix all ingredients together. Pour into greased 9 × 13 inch pan. Bake at 350 degrees for 45 minutes. Let cool before cutting into bars.

Serves 6–8.

Power Balls

These are tasty and extremely dense packets of nutrition. Peanut butter has a nearly universal appeal to children. These are ideal whenever you need a blast of energy. If weight is a concern, use non-fat dried milk. It will supply all the calcium and protein of whole milk with fewer calories.

Ingredients:

1 cup creamy peanut butter
¼ cup dried green leaf powder or leaf concentrate
¼ cup raisins
¼ cup powdered milk
¼ cup sweetened shredded coconut

Directions:

Knead all the ingredients except the shredded coconut together by hand. Roll this mixture into balls 1–1½ inches in diameter. Spread coconut on a cookie sheet or plate, and roll the balls in the coconut until they are evenly coated. Good for 2 days without refrigeration or 2 weeks with it.

Makes about 15 power balls.

Shiso Pesto

Traditional pesto, or pesto Genovese, is made with basil and pine nuts. An interesting variation of pesto can be made by replacing basil with the leaves of shiso (Perilla frutescens), a closely related aromatic plant in the mint family. Shiso adds an exotic flavor that is very popular in Japan.

Ingredients:

1½ cups fresh shiso leaves, removed from stems

¼ cup fresh parsley

2 cloves garlic, crushed

¼ cup chopped walnuts or pine nuts

½ cup grated Parmesan cheese

¼ cup olive oil

½ lb dry pasta

Directions:

Blend all ingredients except pasta in a food processor until a smooth paste is formed. Cook pasta until tender. Toss pesto with hot drained pasta.

Serves 2–3.

Note: In place of or basil or shiso you might also try using another Japanese favorite, garland chrysanthemum (*Chrysanthemum coronarium*). Cilantro, Okinawa spinach, and toon are other flavorful greens that can be used in pesto. You can also substitute walnuts, almonds, or peanuts for pricey pine nuts. Fresh pesto can add a luxurious touch to any pasta, rice, or potato dish.

Extra pesto can be frozen in an ice cube tray to make convenient portions for later use. Pesto is delicious, but packs a lot of calories.

Stuffed Grape Leaves

Ingredients:

1 medium onion, chopped

2 medium tomatoes, chopped

1½ cups cooked spinach, quail grass,
   or young cowpea leaves, chopped

½ tsp salt

½ tsp black pepper

1 cup uncooked rice

1 tsp of lemon juice

Large leaves to use as wrappers.
   Grape leaves are traditional.
   Walking stick kale, Swiss chard,
   chaya, or napa cabbage leaves can
   also be used.

Directions:

Soften wrapping leaves in a bowl of hot water.

Mix all other ingredients together in a large bowl. Place some of the mixture on a leaf. Fold both longer edges of leaf toward the center. Then roll from the stem end toward the top to seal ingredients inside. When all leaves are filled, layer them in a pot. Add enough water to cover leaf layers. Add a few drops of oil and lemon juice to the water to reduce discoloration. Cover and bring to a boil. Lower heat and cook 1–1½ hours until most of the water has been absorbed.

Serves 4–6.

PART IV

Looking Ahead

15

Open-Source Gardening

❊ ❊ ❊

A New Way to Share Information about Food

Globally, the price of most foods has been rising significantly for at least the past 30 years. The prices of basic grains (wheat, rice, and corn) roughly tripled from 1980 to 2012. The price of high-quality food produced with environmentally responsible methods has risen even more. So far, the incomes of the fortunate among us have risen enough to offset the increasing cost of food. However, as wages stagnate and unemployment and underemployment threaten, many more families are beginning to feel squeezed by rising food prices.

The main reason the price of food has increased is that the price of the things needed to produce food (or agricultural inputs) has gone up. As farmers were shaving their labor costs to the bone, the price of farmland, gasoline, fertilizer, and seeds all tripled. The only important agricultural input that has resisted the rising price tide is information.

Advances in computer technology and the development of the Internet have made access to information dramatically faster, cheaper, and more democratic than ever before. To put this in perspective, consider that while other inputs were tripling in price, the cost of storing or transmitting 1,000 pages of text now costs next to nothing. In 1980, I paid $10 per page to fax a letter overseas.

When I began working on agriculture and nutrition issues in the 1970s, I would often have to drive to the National Agriculture Library outside Washington, DC, to get information. That impressive library was (and still is) open only from 8:30 to 4:30, Monday through Friday (same hours as maximum rush-hour traffic). Now, I can quickly search for information from considerably larger databases from the comfort of my home in rural eastern Kentucky. This online "library" is conveniently open 24 hours a day, seven days a week. Using it is also much faster than rummaging through Dewey decimal stacks. For example, typing in the search string "toxins in cassava leaves," I am rewarded with three million results in a small fraction of a second. Not all of these hits are useful, of course, but the first few hundred probably have some relevance to the subject.

It is not just researchers sifting through esoteric studies that benefit from this new worldwide library.

Quick access to information enables beginning gardeners to quickly learn how to make raised planting beds or a trellis or a cabbage moth repellent. A growing segment of this library is available as instructional video clips that walk beginners step-by-step through new techniques.

With access being so cheap and so fast, the number of Internet users has grown rapidly. As of June 2012, there were over 2.4 billion people worldwide using the Internet. This is roughly six times the number of people who were connected to it in 2000. As this new tool moves unprecedented volumes of data around the world, two distinct modes for sharing that information are becoming dominant. These are the *intellectual property model* and the *open-source model*.

Intellectual Property

Intellectual property is a legal concept that gives exclusive or monopoly rights to mental creations such as inventions, designs, music, art, and software for a certain period of time. Patents, copyrights, and trademarks are common tools used for defining and enforcing intellectual property rights. The primary justification for intellectual property laws is that they establish incentives for people to do creative work that benefits society as a whole. At least in theory, they allow a means of rewarding inventive thinkers—and preventing others from stealing the fruit of that thinking. While there is general agreement that financial reward can be a motivator, it is less clear how much reward is needed to motivate. Will a person be 1,000 times more creative for a billion dollars than for a million dollars?

In practice, things quickly get even murkier because information is not like furniture or sandwiches. If someone transfers a sandwich to you (you're correct if you guessed it's almost lunch time as I write this), they are left without it. However, if they transfer an idea to you, they can still retain that idea, so now both have it. Idea transfer is not a zero-sum game, like sandwich transfer. Intellectual property is inherently nebulous because ideas comingle readily, and it is frequently unclear where one idea stops and another one starts. Here, one enters the fantastic realm of patent infringement law with all of its posturing, preemptive threatening, and multi-million dollar settlements.

Many critics believe that intellectual property rights create artificial scarcity by withholding useful knowledge from people who are unable to pay. They suggest that the free flow of information is the lifeblood of a modern economy and that minimizing intellectual property rights would reduce some of the bottlenecks that are currently impeding that flow.

Open-Source

Open-source is a relatively new approach to information sharing that differs sharply from the dominant intellectual property rights model. The Internet itself is basically a shared open-source tool that provides the backbone for the Information Age. The term "open-source" was first popularized in 1998 when the source code for the Navigator Internet browser was made freely available to the public. Originally a new system for developing and distributing computer software, the principles of open-source are now being extended, with myriad variations, to designing farm machinery, modular housing, solar electric equipment, automobiles, college textbooks, washing machines, and pharmaceuticals. The open-source concept is quickly spreading to university courses, music sharing, and travel arranging, among many other areas.

At the core of open-source development are the communities of peers that connect with each other, usually through the Internet, in order to work together on a common project. In an open-source community, participants contribute to, as well as benefit from, shared information or content. Members of the community (and usually the public at large) are encouraged to reproduce, modify, and redistribute open-source information, building on the work of other people and sharing the benefit of the collaboration. All of this generally happens without the end users of the information incurring any financial cost.

In a culture nearly obsessed with the virtues of ownership and market capitalism, this may sound a bit like the addled idealistic rambling of hippies. Open-source should be easily flicked away by the pragmatic and realistic people who run our economy. It would be, except that it seems to work. Probably the most famous example of an open-source contribution to our society is Wikipedia. This online encyclopedia began in 2001, and was written via the collaboration of thousands of unpaid and generally anonymous volunteers. By 2012 it had become the largest encyclopedia in history, with over 77,000 active contributors working on over 22,000,000 articles in 285 languages. Its website is visited by roughly 470 million people each month.

Open-source is especially well suited to projects like software or pharmaceuticals or seed development, where the product is fundamentally information. Typically it requires a great deal of time, effort, and money to develop original codes, or formulas, or genetics. However, reproducing the software, drugs, or seeds is often very cheap. In the case of software, the most developed part of the open-source economy, it is essentially free. (Incidentally, this book was written with Ubuntu and Libre Office free open-source software.) Reproducing drugs is a bit more complex, but still certainly possible. When South Africa threatened to replicate expensive patented drugs in order to treat millions of people with AIDS, drug companies quickly slashed their prices and went to court to protect their monopolies.

When most of us think about software and drugs, we envision disks and pills. We may think of seeds as tiny objects that we plant, but Monsanto thinks of seeds as genetic formulas over which they can gain exclusive control. This is the Age of Information, and now most of that economic value in those industries is in the monopoly control of that information. It is no accident that the wealthiest individuals and most profitable corporations are the gate-keepers of information. Some of that guarded information could improve the lives of countless people were it distributed more freely and at a greatly lower price. Open-source is an interesting challenge to an outdated economic model on behalf of the world's low-income people.

Much of the criticism of the open-source movement focuses on the issues of stability and reliability. How can an information system that is continually open to anonymous input from the public provide a stable working environment? How can it guarantee that the malicious or misinformed won't corrupt the information?

Open-Sourcing the Garden

Nowhere is the contrast between the open-source world view and the intellectual property perspective greater than in food and agriculture. The poster child for intellectual property in the food system is Monsanto, the world's biggest seed company. They own patents on engineered plant genetics and jealously guard this secret information. The company makes much of its money not by producing seeds but by controlling access to genetic information that would allow farmers to easily produce their own seeds. They have repeatedly sued their own customers for patent infringement. These are usually farmers who engaged in the time-honored, but in this case illegal, practice of saving seed to plant the following year.

The big biotechnology firms inhabit a world of valuable secrets. They not only keep their genetic secrets from the farmers who buy their seeds, they lobby furiously to keep the public from even knowing whether or not they are consuming their genetically modified foods. The big food companies have systematically resisted every effort, such as nutritional labeling, to inform the public about the food they are being sold.

Open-source communities, on the other hand, have little use for expensive secrets. This is as true with home gardeners as with software users. The emergence of low-cost and high-speed access to information combined with the enormous pool of Internet users is especially relevant to home gardeners. Uniting the global sweep of the Internet with the intimately local and pragmatic kitchen garden creates dynamic opportunities for both the gardeners and for the growth of the open-source strategy. Gardeners can have their eyes opened to a wide world of horticultural experience. At the same time, the real-life concerns of people, their plants, and their food can help ground the far-flung domain of open-source enthusiasts.

Open-source gardening can function at various scales. If the multinational biotechnology corporations occupy one end of the agricultural information spectrum, the other extreme is the rapidly growing phenomenon of local seed libraries. Often based in public libraries, these are free exchanges of garden seeds. Generally, one can "borrow" seeds for the plant-ing season, and return seeds that have been carefully saved from the harvest. In this way, gardeners can save money on seeds, begin developing locally adapted varieties, and share their experiences with other local gardeners.

There are also several Internet-based seed exchanges with wider geo-graphical range that generally adhere to open-source principles. These in-clude the large and well-established Seed Savers Exchange (seedsavers.org), as well as numerous newer and smaller garden seed networks, such as The Seed Commons (seedmatters.org) and the Open Source Seed Bank (sites .google.com/site/ossbank). These groups are often focused on preserving the genetic heritage of our heirloom crops as commonly held wealth.

Another exciting approach to open-source agriculture comes from the Cambia Foundation and other groups that are working to meld the gene mapping of biotechnology with traditional plant breeding methods. Rather than directly manipulating the plants genetics by inserting foreign genes, they seek to use sophisticated gene maps to help visualize and arrange har-monious crosses of varieties. This could greatly increase the speed and ac-curacy of traditional plant breeding and reduce the cost of developing stable crop varieties better adapted to specific climates, pests, diseases, and soil types. Importantly, the results of this work generally cannot be patented and can be freely reproduced by farmers and gardeners.

The open-source approach to information sharing is nearly a perfect match for the social structure of home gardening. There are millions of kitchen gardeners who share a common interest in growing good food and have little motive for manipulating each other. While the commercial food system is driven largely by the linear math of return on investment (ROI), the world of home gardening runs on more complex and socially integrated motivations. The diminished role of financial reward reduces competition and enables the home gardening movement to make better use of coopera-tive open-source strategies. Kitchen gardeners are well positioned to benefit from low-cost information sharing networks.

Here is an example: There are over 90,000 local governments in the US and Canada. Many, if not most, of them have ordinances controlling the rights to keep chickens or to have a front yard vegetable garden. Many of these regulations are antiquated, vague, or arbitrarily enforced. As interest in home food production grows, the number of conflicts over these local ordinances is also increasing rapidly. An open-source database that organizes these laws and the outcomes of conflicts they've produced would help a gardener in Arkansas access the similar experiences of gardeners in California or Delaware to help assert her right to grow a vegetable patch.

There has already been some success with this strategy. The municipal council in Drummondville, Quebec, reversed its decision to force the removal of a front yard vegetable garden after they received a petition with 29,000 signatures. The petition was initiated by Kitchen Garden International and distributed through Causes.com, a website that "provides free and easy tools for passionate people to spread the word, find supporters, raise money, and build momentum."

There are many benefits from open-sourcing gardening—access to locally adapted seeds; rototiller sharing; advance warning of changes in pest or pollinator populations; designs and feedback for do-it-yourself garden tools, trellises, cold frames, and planting beds; and recipes and food preservation techniques are among the many possibilities. For gardeners, open-source probably won't help with shoveling manure or hoeing weeds, but it could be very useful in finding out who has manure to shovel or which weed is invading the garden.

A dynamic interface between home gardening and the open-source world is rapidly evolving with the advent of simple, low-cost robotic hardware. For example, Arduino and Raspberry Pi are producing thousands of micro-computers designed for robotic tinkering that sell for less than $50. The size of a pack of cards, they run open-source software and are being programmed by our gum-chewing tattooed youth to monitor soil moisture and automatically water garden crops.

Free access to practical horticultural information increases the yield of fruits and vegetables that home gardeners can harvest. The gap between what an average gardener harvests and what top gardeners can bring to the table is enormous. The cutting-edge techniques of top vegetable gardeners are percolating through the World Wide Web, and a generation of young kitchen gardeners are quickly closing that gap. The work of John Jeavons of Ecology Action, the Dervaes family of Homegrown Revolution, Eric Toensmeier of Perennial Solutions, and of the British horticulturist Joy Larkcom, as well as dozens of other inspiring gardeners, are enabling kitchen gardeners to grow much more high-quality food in smaller areas.

Ready access to accurate information benefits all growers, but the minimal cost of open-source information is especially important for low-income home gardeners. Learning how to grow the most nutritious foods, either at home or in a community garden, can improve the diet and health of low-income families while making minimal demands on their scarce cash. Encouragingly, use of the Internet is increasing the fastest among low-income households, those that could most benefit from more productive home kitchen gardens. As an extreme example, in sub-Saharan Africa, the poorest region on Earth—and not coincidently the area with the highest rates of malnutrition—the number of Internet users has been increasing by 45 percent a year since 2005.[1]

No King of the Jungle

Lions rely on the bacteria in soil to make nutrients available to the grasses that feed the antelopes they eat. Lions die and are eaten by buzzards and the bacteria that feed the grass. There is no king of the jungle. Much of the power and the potential of open-source gardening networks stems from the fact that they resemble natural ecosystems more closely than do the traditional hierarchies that dominate our business, government, and military affairs.

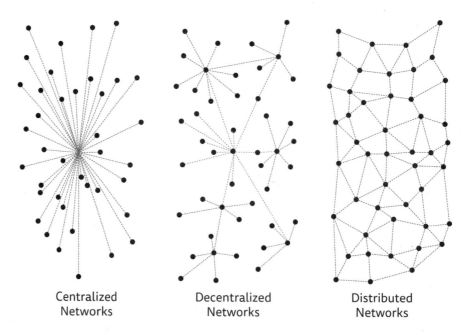

Centralized
Networks

Decentralized
Networks

Distributed
Networks

Having a large pool of participants with minimal financial motivation gives open-source networks the same sort of checks and balances that enable ecosystems to function. Open-source systems like Wikipedia, with transparent structures, high-speed information exchange, a large number of participants, and lack of personal financial motive, are remarkably good at managing massive amounts of data and quickly correcting false information. This ability to organically self-regulate and self-heal gives open-source systems a huge advantage over closed systems.

Open-source systems are noticeably free from the inundation of advertisements that plague our culture. They inherently lack the incentives to dis-inform people. Systems run smoother with better information. While our political systems seem to be stagnating into gridlock, open-source offers something new. An efficient means of generating wealth that requires neither government funding nor government regulation is a win-win for the small-government people. At the same time, a radically democratic means of more equitably sharing wealth and power is appealing to social justice supporters.

Open-source strategies allow many anonymous volunteer contributors to create something truly great. The highly dispersed nature of open-source networks matches the demographics and financial motivation of home gardeners perfectly. Open-source gardening can access the creativity of millions of people, greatly improving the yield, quality, and distribution of the most local of foods. Open-source is new and surely experiencing some growing pains, but its potential to improve our food system is enormous.

I feel strongly that the last word in economics
is open source economics....
It is called sharing.

« Marcin Jakubowski »
director of Open Source Ecology,
opensourceecology.org

16

Growing Home

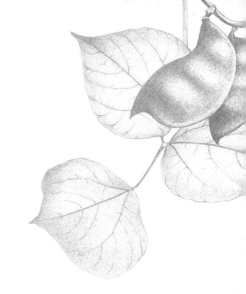

❈ ❈ ❈

Held in the Light

Sitting out in the garden on a sunny early spring day, my skin soaks up the energy in the sunlight so that chemicals in my skin can make the vitamin D my body needs. Next to me, a kale stretches out so that chemicals in its leaves can catch the sunlight and make the carbohydrates it needs. I look at the world around me. Lutein and beta-carotene help my eyes process light and protect them from the damaging ultraviolet rays of the sun. I get my lutein and beta-carotene from my dark green kale plants. They use lutein and beta-carotene to process light and protect their leaves from the damaging ultraviolet rays of the sun. I keep the kale plants healthy with compost, mulch, and water. I take care of them. They take care of me. What a team!

For over 40 years, I have been growing greens in kitchen gardens and have teamed up with a lot of plants. For 30 of those years, I have also served as the director of Leaf for Life, a non-profit organization that combats malnutrition in the tropics. We focus on making better use of leaf crops because they can resolve many common nutritional problems with little cash investment. They are especially good for reducing iron deficiency anemia and vitamin A deficiency, two of the world's most common health problems.

Green leaves are also remarkably good at addressing the world's fastest growing type of malnutrition: obesity. Leaf vegetables provide the vitamins, minerals, and antioxidants that are most promising in fighting obesity (and the common degenerative diseases that accompany it), with the fewest calories of any foods.

We need to find low-cost ways to resolve these two very different types of nutritional problems. The consequences of leaving both types unchecked are intolerably expensive. Furthermore, we need to solve current nutritional problems without damaging food-producing land. We can't forget that people will still need food in the future.

Reducing both types of malnutrition while trying to protect natural environments is a big job. Way too big. About two billion people, six times the population of the entire US, suffer from anemia (low levels of iron in their blood). Half a million kids go blind every year from lack of vitamin A. Over one billion people are now overweight or obese. At the same time, 850 million people go to bed hungry most nights. Some of us need more food, and all of us need better food, but producing more food is already polluting our water, turning grasslands into deserts, and emptying the oceans of fish.

Your eyes are glazing over! I don't blame you. It wears on us being continually reminded and warned about dangers that we have little control over. Some of the most vexing and persistent warnings pertain to the threats of global environmental degradation and food shortages. That these two dangers appear to be intricately entwined makes things seem even more threatening.

We are warned repeatedly of the dangers of too many parts per million of carbon in our air, and of billions of tons of topsoil eroding, and of our governments owing trillions of dollars. It's been over 200 years since Thomas Malthus warned us that a growing population would eventually outrun its food supply. Over 50 years ago, Rachel Carson wrote *Silent Spring*, warning us of grave environmental consequences from the overuse of agricultural chemicals. About 25 years ago, the UN began warning us of the catastrophic changes in climate patterns to come unless we immediately changed our carbon-spewing ways.

We are much better adapted to reacting to acute short-term threats than we are at dealing with gradually intensifying danger. We have been warned—and we are growing numb to the warnings. Putting the warnings in larger fonts with more exclamation points probably won't help much.

We are not very good at imagining, much less acting quickly and rationally on, information that is wildly outside the scope and scale of our personal physical existence. We know about atoms from school, but have a hard time visualizing a solid steel ball-bearing as almost entirely empty space between the atomic nuclei and the rings of orbiting electrons. We see stars in the night sky, and are told that the light we see has been traveling across space at 186,000 *miles* a second, but we describe a baseball thrown at 150 *feet* a second as a "blazing" fastball. And it really strains our brains to hear that some of those night stars that we are looking directly at ceased to exist long before the rise and fall of the Roman Empire. We are a species of primates that learned to count with our fingers not so very long ago. We are stupefied and overwhelmed by vastness.

When we read that we will need to double food production in order to feed the 9 billion hungry people we expect to be alive in 2050, what does it mean? Can you visualize a line of pick-up trucks loaded with food stretching bumper-to-bumper from New York to Los Angeles and back seven times to supply just one day's worth of food? I can't. Like most people, I am completely freaked out by even a five-mile long-traffic jam.

No one wants people to go hungry. No one wants birds or frogs or elephants to become extinct. No one wants the natural world to collapse around us. Seeing a young child dying from the lack of food is the most heart-wrenching experience imaginable, but for most of us the hungry masses are hungry somewhere far away. Most of us rarely see farms anymore, much less the chemicals used on them. We can't see, smell, or touch the carbon dioxide in the air, and the weather has always seemed unpredictable.

Maybe half of us suspect there truly is an impending ecological apocalypse, but few really feel it. It is not the visceral sort of fear that comes from a door creaking open in the middle of the night. Increasingly, we love Nature in the same way that we fear its doom: abstractly, and from a distance. A stroll through a tree-lined park, a weekend camping trip, signing petitions, recycling cans—these are the trappings of a respectful, platonic love.

Most people would like to rise to the occasion, making sure everyone has enough to eat and that the ecological systems that food production depends on are well protected. Who really wants to be remembered as the generation that let the future die? But what to do? These are global issues, and they require grand and well-funded schemes from big players like the UN, national governments, universities, and foundations. We will also need a few dazzlingly brilliant creative ideas from the next wave of Nobel Prize candidates.

Most people don't work for UNICEF or stand a shot at winning a Nobel Prize. Most of us need to work with bite-sized pieces of the world in order to not feel overwhelmed by the task. For most people, a home kitchen garden is a manageable-sized piece of the world. Something that can be measured with paces and counted with fingers.

Unlike a planet, a plant can be loved in a physical and intimate way, and the best gardeners are in love. They caress the Earth, suffer with the droughts, and thrill to the labors of sprouting seeds breaking the soil's crust and taking their first taste of sunshine. They feed the garden with the leftovers of their lives, and eat what the garden yields to them.

While the big institutions are grappling with the big issues, the time is ripe for the legions of home gardeners to step up their game and create millions of micro-Edens. We need more hands in the dirt, more muscle and sweat. There are small places everywhere waiting for stouthearted gardeners willing to do the hard work of rejuvenating damaged land. The garden is a place, however small it may be, that one can keep making better. It is a refuge from the superficial, where we can sit in peaceful solidarity with the sun and the leaves. The humble home garden offers the average person the chance to stand against the looming catastrophe and actually heal and protect a small part of the natural world. To leave a place more beautiful and productive, more vibrant and full of life than you found it, this is the honorable work—and the endless task of recreating earthly paradise.

Why do we need so many kinds of apples?
Because there are so many folks....
There is merit in variety itself.
It provides more points of contact with life,
and leads away from uniformity and monotony.

« LIBERTY HYDE BAILEY »

Appendix 1: Seeds and Supplies

Agro Haitai: Canadian-based source for reasonably priced Asian vegetable seeds.
agrohaitai.com

B & T World Seeds: French-based company with one of the largest collections of unusual vegetable seeds in the world.
b-and-t-world-seeds.com

Bountiful Gardens: Vegetable seeds and legume inoculants. Excellent gardening information from bio-intensive perspective.
bountifulgardens.org

Chiltern Seeds: British-based company with very large selection of vegetable seeds.
chilternseeds.co.uk

Evergreen Seeds: 350 varieties of Asian vegetable seeds and books for Oriental gardening and cooking.
evergreenseeds.com/vegetableseeds.html

Fedco Seeds: Good, inexpensive garden seeds and an informative catalog.
fedcoseeds.com

Florida Herb House: Sells dried spinach and alfalfa.
sharpweblabs.com

Frontier Natural Products Coop: Sells a variety of dried vegetable powders.
frontiercoop.com

Growers Supply: A large selection of greenhouse and other commercial agriculture supplies at good prices. Based in Louisiana.
growersupply.com

Johnny's Selected Seeds: Large selection of organic and non-organic vegetable seeds, especially for cooler climates; garden supplies and informative catalog.
johnnyseeds.com

Kitazawa Seed Company: US company specializing in Asian vegetable seeds.
kitazawaseed.com

Mass Spectrum Botanicals: Tampa, Florida-based company with many unusual leaf crop seeds and plants.
massspectrumbotanicals.com

Nichols Garden Nursery: Family-owned source of seed for many unusual leaf vegetables.
nicholsgardennursery.com

Nuts.com: Family-owned source of dried moringa and wheatgrass.

Peaceful Valley Farm Supply: Very large selection of organic seeds and supplies, including good range of cover crop seeds and agricultural tools; geared toward organic farms and larger gardens.
groworganic.com

Pinetree Garden Seeds: Good selection of inexpensive vegetable seed in small packets.
superseeds.com

Sakata Seeds: Japanese seed company with distributors throughout the world.
sakata.com

Seeds of India: New Jersey company specializing in vegetable seeds of the Indian sub-continent.
seedsofindia.com

Terroir Seeds: Arizona-based company specializing in heirloom vegetable seed.
underwoodgardens.com

Thompson & Morgan Seeds: British company with huge selection of vegetable seeds. Has a US and a Canadian branch.
thompson-morgan.com

Z Natural Foods: Sells dried moringa, barley, alfalfa, spinach, and other dried leaf powders.
znaturalfoods.com

Appendix 2: Useful Websites

American Community Gardening Association: Support for the community garden movement in the United States and Canada with much useful vegetable gardening information.
communitygarden.org

Association for the Promotion of Leaf Concentrate in Nutrition: Information on the production and consumption of leaf concentrate, especially from alfalfa, for the alleviation of malnutrition in English and French.
nutrition-luzerne.org/anglais/index2.htm

Center for New Crops & Plant Products: Information on new and specialty crops.
hort.purdue.edu/newcrop

Educational Concerns for Hunger Organization (ECHO): Site contains a wealth of information on unusual leaf crops.
echonet.org

Food and Nutrition Information Center (FNIC): Mainstream nutrition information from the US National Agriculture Library including extensive composition of foods databases.
fnic.nal.usda.gov

Kitchen Gardeners International: A network of over 30,000 people from 100 countries promoting greater food self-reliance through home vegetable gardens.
kitchengardeners.org

Leaf for Life: Information on making better use of leaf crops to improve human nutrition, especially leaf concentrate and dried leaf powders.
leafforlife.org

Moringanews: An international network linking people working with moringa and providing excellent non-commercial information on the various uses of this plant.
moringanews.org

National Sustainable Agriculture Information Service: Publications on sustainable production practices, alternative crops, and innovative marketing.
attra.ncat.org/index.php

Plants For A Future: Information on ecologically sustainable horticulture including a database of approximately 7,000 edible species and otherwise useful plants.
pfaf.org

Plant Physiology Online: A well-organized collection of essays covering all aspects of plant physiology, mainly on a college level.
4e.plantphys.net/contents.php

Plant Resources of Tropical Africa: Extensive information on roughly 7,000 useful African plants, including many unusual leaf vegetables.
prota.org

The International Seed Saving Institute: Basic seed saving information on saving seeds with specific instructions for 27 vegetables.
seedsave.org

World Vegetable Center (formerly the Asian Vegetable Research and Development Center): Excellent source of information on leaf crops, especially Asian leaf crops.
avrdc.org

Notes

Introduction
1. Food Marketing Institute, fmi.org
2. USDA Agricultural Marketing Service, 08/03/2012.

Chapter 1
1. Bittman, Mark. "California's Central Valley, Land of a Billion Vegetables," *The New York Times Magazine*, October 10, 2012, nytimes.com
2. "The Average American Ate (Literally) a Ton This Year," (compiled from USDA's Economic Research Service data, 2011), npr.org
3. "Society at a Glance 2011: OECD Social Indicators," oecd.org
4. National Restaurant Association, "Restaurant Industry Pocket Facts Book," restaurant.org
5. Hall, Kevin D., Juen Guo, Michael Dore, and Carson C. Chow. "The Progressive Increase of Food Waste in America and Its Environmental Impact." PLoS ONE 4, no. 11 (November 25, 2009).
6. Blanco-Canqui, Humberto, and R. Lal. *Principles of Soil Conservation and Management*. Springer, 2008, page 11.
7. Siebert, Charles. "Food Ark," *National Geographic* 220 (2011): 108–131.
8. Fowler, Cary, and Patrick R. Mooney. *Shattering: Food, Politics, and the Loss of Genetic Diversity*. University of Arizona Press, 1990, page 63.
9. "FASTSTATS: Overweight Prevalence," 2014. Accessed January 23, 2014. cdc.gov
10. Cawley, John, and Chad Meyerhoefer. 2012. "The Medical Care Costs of Obesity: An Instrumental Variables Approach," *Journal of Health Economics* 31 (1): 219–30.
11. American Diabetes Association. 2013. "Economic Costs of Diabetes in the U.S. in 2012." *Diabetes Care* 36 (4): 1033–46.

Chapter 2
1. Swenson, Paulina. "Paired Price Comparisons of Farmers' Market and Supermarket Produce in San Luis Obispo County," *Agribusiness* March 1, 2012. digitalcommons.calpoly.edu
2. Drewnowski, Adam. "The Cost of US Foods As Related to Their Nutritive Value," *The American Journal of Clinical Nutrition* 92, no. 5 (November 1, 2010): 1181–1188.

3. Carlson, Andi, and Elizabeth Frazao. "Are Healthy Foods Really More Expensive? It Depends on How You Measure the Price," Rochester, NY: Social Science Research Network, January 18, 2013. papers.ssrn.com

4. Shrestha, Ishani. "Can Community Supported Agriculture be an Economically Viable Approach to Sustainable Agriculture?" December 17, 2012, ida.mtholyoke.edu

5. Paarlberg Robert. "The Culture War over Food and Farming: Who is Winning?" University of Wisconsin, April 20, 2012, aae.wisc.edu

6. *The Economist* "Special Report: Food Politics—Voting with Your Trolley," December 9, 2006, economist.com

7. ibid.

8. Roper, Natalie. "SNAP Redemptions at Farmers Markets Exceed $11 Million in 2011," Posted January 18th, 2012, farmersmarketcoalition.org

Chapter 3

1. Bruce Butterfield, National Gardening Association Research Director, "The Impact of Home and Community Gardening In America" 2009, National Gardening Association: South Burlington, VT.

2. ibid.

3. Alaimo, K., et al. "Fruit and Vegetable Intake Among Urban Community Gardeners," *J Nutr Educ Behav* 2008, Mar-Apr 40(2): 94–101.

4. Langellotto, Gail A., and Abha Gupta. "Gardening Increases Vegetable Consumption in School-aged Children: A Meta-analytical Synthesis," Department of Horticulture, Oregon State University.

Chapter 4

1. Stuart, Tristram. *Waste: Uncovering the Global Food Scandal*. New York: W. W. Norton & Co., 2009.

2. Wells, Hodan Farah, and Jean C. Buzby. "Dietary Assessment of Major Trends in US Food Consumption, 1970–2005." US Department of Agriculture, Economic Research Service, 2008. ers.usda.gov

Chapter 5

1. Scientific American, "For a Healthier Country, Overhaul Farm Subsidies," Accessed January 31, 2013. scientificamerican.com

2. Goran, Michael I., Stanley J. Ulijaszek, and Emily E. Ventura. "High Fructose Corn Syrup and Diabetes Prevalence: A Global Perspective," *Global Public Health* 2013, 8(1): 55–66.

3. Carter, P., L. J. Gray, J. Troughton, K. Khunti, and M. J. Davies. "Fruit and Vegetable Intake and Incidence of Type 2 Diabetes Mellitus: Systematic Review and Meta-analysis." *BMJ* 341, (August, 2010): c4229–c4229.

4. "CDC: Attribution of Foodborne Illness, 1998–2008—Estimates of Foodborne Illness." cdc.gov/foodborneburden

5. Kozak, G. K., et al., "Foodborne Outbreaks in Canada Linked to Produce: 2001 through 2009." *Journal of Food Protection* 76, no. 1 (2013): 173–183.
6. "Executive Summary: Eat Your Fruits and Vegetables!" Environmental Working Group. Accessed February 1, 2013. ewg.org

Chapter 6

1. The temperate zone refers to the part of the earth between the Tropic of Cancer and the Arctic Circle in the Northern Hemisphere or between the Tropic of Capricorn and the Antarctic Circle in the Southern Hemisphere. Typically, land in the temperate zone has a climate that is warm in the summer, cold in the winter, and moderate in the spring and fall. *The tropics* refers formally to the part of the earth between the latitudes of 23½ degrees north and 23½ degrees south. Because of the tilt in the polar axis, this part of the earth has the sun directly overhead at least once a year. In popular usage, the tropics is the part of the world where it is warm year-round and seldom freezes.
2. "2011 Community Preference Survey." 2014. Realtor.org. Accessed February 2, 2014. realtor.org
3. Whiting, D. with C. O'Meara, and C. Carl Wilson. "Block Style Layout in Raised Bed Vegetable Gardens." CMG GardenNotes #713, Colorado Master Gardener Program Yard and Garden Publications, 2012, ext.colostate.edu
4. The pH scale is used for measuring acidity. It runs from 0 to 14, with 7 representing neutral or distilled water. Lower numbers indicate increasing acidity, and higher numbers mean increasing alkalinity. A soil pH of 6.3–6.8 is considered optimal for the availability of plant nutrients.
5. tanksforless.com
6. "How Bacteria in Our Bodies Protect Our Health." Accessed August 4, 2013. scientificamerican.com

Chapter 7

1. Kuti, J. O. and E. S. Torres. 1996. "Potential Nutritional and Health Benefits of Tree Spinach." In: J. Janick (ed.), *Progress in New Crops*. ASHS Press: Arlington, VA, 516–520.
2. "Moringa Leaf Extract As a Plant Growth Hormone," ECHO Development Note 68, June 2000, echonet.org

Chapter 9

1. Mellinger, A. D., J. D. Sachs, and J. L. Gallup. "Climate, Water Navigability, and Economic Development," Working Paper. University of Chicago Graduate School of Business, 2000. econpapers.repec.org
2. Coleman, Eliot. *The Winter Harvest Handbook: Year-Round Vegetable Production Using Deep-Organic Techniques and Unheated Greenhouses*. 2009. Chelsea Green Publishing, page 44.

3. Coleman, *The Winter Harvest Handbook*, page 3.
4. Organic Farming Research Foundation Project Report, "Shade-Covered High Tunnels for Summer Production of Lettuce and Leafy Greens," Katherine Kelly, Full Circle Farm, Kansas City, Kansas, ofrf.org

Chapter 15

1. Nisbet, Erik C., Elizabeth Stoycheff, and Katy E. Pearce. "Internet Use and Democratic Demands: A Multinational, Multilevel Model of Internet Use and Citizen Attitudes About Democracy," *Journal of Communication* 62.2 (2012): 249–265.

Index

Page numbers in **bold** indicate main discussion of plant.

About the Illustrator

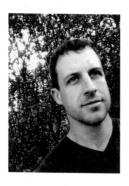

KEITH WILDE is a freelance artist, illustrator, and art educator living in Athens, Ohio. Keith has exhibited his art across the nation and won numerous awards. Some of his recent illustration talent can be seen in *Leaf for Life Handbook*, by David Kennedy, and in art direction for *Moose on the Loose*, by Kim Kerns, a children's book illustrated by his students. keithwilde.com

About the Author

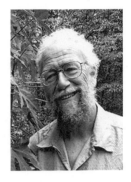

DAVE KENNEDY is the founder and director of Leaf for Life, a nonprofit organization dedicated to the elimination of global malnutrition through the optimum use of leaf crops to support human health. He has designed and implemented projects and workshops involving small-scale agriculture and innovative food processing in 13 different countries on four continents. The author of *21st Century Greens* and the *Leaf for Life Handbook*, David is a tireless advocate for the development of wholesome food systems worldwide.

If you have enjoyed *Eat Your Greens*, you might also enjoy other

BOOKS TO BUILD A NEW SOCIETY

Our books provide positive solutions for people who
want to make a difference. We specialize in:

Sustainable Living ◆ Green Building ◆ Peak Oil
Renewable Energy ◆ Environment & Economy
Natural Building & Appropriate Technology
Progressive Leadership ◆ Resistance and Community
Educational & Parenting Resources

New Society Publishers

ENVIRONMENTAL BENEFITS STATEMENT

New Society Publishers has chosen to produce this book on recycled paper made
with 100% post consumer waste, processed chlorine free, and old growth free.

For every 5,000 books printed, New Society saves the following resources:[1]

37	Trees
3,391	Pounds of Solid Waste
3,731	Gallons of Water
4,866	Kilowatt Hours of Electricity
6,164	Pounds of Greenhouse Gases
27	Pounds of HAPs, VOCs, and AOX Combined
9	Cubic Yards of Landfill Space

---

[1]Environmental benefits are calculated based on research done by the Environmental Defense Fund and
other members of the Paper Task Force who study the environmental impacts of the paper industry.

For a full list of NSP's titles, please call 1-800-567-6772 or check out our web site at:

www.newsociety.com

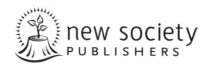

new society
PUBLISHERS